Poisoning Our Children

Surviving in a Toxic World

Nancy Sokol Green

The Noble Press, Inc.

Copyright 1991 by Nancy Sokol Green. All rights reserved.

No part of this book may be reproduced or transmitted in any form or by any means, electronic or mechanical, including photocopying, recording or by any information storage and retrieval system, without written permission from the publisher.

Printed in the United States of America

Library of Congress Cataloging-in-Publication Data

Green, Nancy Sokol
Poisoning our children : surviving in a toxic world / Nancy Sokol Green
p. cm.
Includes bibliographical references and index
ISBN 0-9622683-7-2 : $12.95
1. Environmentally induced diseases. 2. Environmental health. 3. Toxicology. I. Title
RA566.G74 1991
616.9'8--dc20   90-63429
CIP

The information, recommendations, and opinions expressed herein are based on the author's own experience with and research on multiple chemical sensitivities. In that the author is not medically or technically trained in this area, the information shared in the book should not be construed as medical or professional advice in the area of environmental illness, but as one suf- ferer's long experience with environmental illness. Neither Nancy Green, Dr. Sherry Rogers, nor The Noble Press assumes any responsibility and disclaims any injury or damage resulting from the opinions or recommendations expressed in this book.

Noble Press books are available in bulk at discount prices. Single copies are available prepaid direct from the publisher:

Marketing Director
The Noble Press, Inc.
213 W. Institute Place, Suite 508
Chicago, Illinois 60610

DEDICATION

For all the children
who suffer from behavioral problems
and/or mild to life-threatening health conditions
from environmental exposures.

CONTENTS

Chapter 3
TOXINS—AT HOME, IN THE NEIGHBORHOOD

Chapter 4
WHAT WE REALLY EAT AND DRINK

FOREWORD

Over the last two decades, I have had the opportunity to treat thousands of people who, like myself, have developed environmental illness (EI). How did these people know they had EI? Most of them didn't. They came to us with specific symptoms, such as headaches, an inability to concentrate, unwarranted depression, and chronic fatigue. They came because of chronic sinusitis, asthma, colitis, eczema, arthritis and many other symptoms.

Environmental medicine is a whole philosophy of practicing medicine. In traditional medicine, a physician accumulates a list of symptoms, completes a history and physical examination, and makes a diagnosis from the information. Once he or she has made the diagnosis, the physician automatically prescribes specific drugs and recommends certain surgeries as the only way to control the symptoms. In contrast, physicians in environmental medicine don't really concern themselves with the *name* of the disease. We care more about discovering the *causes* of the affliction, and we now have the tools with which to find many of the environmental factors and biochemical deficiencies that trigger certain reactions—we can now actually get rid of many of the symptoms once and for all *without* drugs.

By the time our patients come to us, many of them have already been to more than a dozen physicians. Many can unfold several feet of computer printouts from their pharmacies showing the drugs that have been prescribed to them by doctors desperate to relieve their symptoms. Eventually, these sufferers realized that drugs could not create health and that they needed to find the underlying causes of their symptoms.

Little wonder their surprise when these patients learned that they were allergic to dusts and molds, intolerant to certain foods, sensitive to Candida and certain chemicals, and deficient in essential nutrients—and that these were the real causes of their symptoms.

Why do people become sensitive to certain chemicals? It is probably because we are the first generation of people ever to have been exposed to so many chemicals. Given the condition of average home or office environments, as well as that of our food and water supplies, the average person is exposed to over 500 chemicals on a daily basis. Some of us are more vulnerable to these chemicals than others.

Normally, the body is able to metabolize and neutralize the chemicals that invade the body. However, when the body is confronted with more chemicals than it can neutralize, it cannot effectively detoxify itself. It's at this point that people get sick.

For every person who displays a reaction to certain chemicals, there are just as many who are able to metabolize or process the chemicals in their bodies and get rid of them efficiently. The biggest obstacle to the body's purging itself of these chemicals efficiently is having too many chemicals vying for the same biochemical detoxification pathways. The situation is made worse when the detoxification system itself is weakened due to a lack of nutrients. (We are, after all, the first generation of people to eat such an unprecedented amount of processed foods.)

Many people who have suffered the devastating effects of chemical sensitivity have remarked that if they had only known that pesticides, home chemicals, processed foods, municipal waters, dental amalgams, and many of the other things that we take for granted had the potential for causing illness, they would have never let themselves become so vulnerable by repeatedly exposing themselves to them.

Many thanks go to Nancy Green for sharing the story of her pesticide poisoning with us so that we might learn from her and for mapping out the important guidelines for detoxifying one's life. Her story is typical of the devastation I have heard from hundreds of others.

Poisoning Our Children will certainly be one of the most helpful books for the American family this decade. Thank you, Nancy, for bringing it to us.

Sherry A. Rogers, M.D., F.A.C.A., A.B.F.P., A.B.E.M.
Northeast Center for Environmental Medicine
2800 West Genesee Street
Syracuse, New York 13219

August, 1991

ACKNOWLEDGMENTS

Without many people there would have been no road to recovery and certainly no book.

I would especially like to thank my parents Marvin and Arline Sokol for their never-ending, unconditional love and support; my daughters Callan and Kiley for all their heart-warming smiles and enormous hugs of encouragement; my grandmother Rebecca Robinson for her unbelievable contribution and special love; my sisters Joanne Sokol and Marcia Harris for their on-going hours of commitment to my family; Mary Strumbos and Julie Carter for their incredible friendship; Nobu and Celine Asano for their extraordinary compassion and expertise in the field of acupuncture; Dr. Ruth Heifetz and Adelia McCord for their invaluable information about environmental illness and toxic chemicals; The Noble Press for their commitment and dedication to my book; and last, but certainly not least, my loving and supportive husband Jim, who was beside me all those long months of darkness—and all the way home.

PREFACE

A few years ago, I could not have even imagined reading a book on chemicals, let alone writing one. After all, my "yuppie" lifestyle did not lend itself to a thorough evaluation of the countless chemicals so intertwined in my life.

Perhaps if I had known then that approximately *seventy thousand* new chemicals have been introduced since World War II, I might have stopped to think about the effects they could have on our everyday lives. But probably not. After all, everyone and everything surrounding me was continually reinforcing my naive perception that the way I was living was safe.

I certainly had never seen any indication of danger on the school grounds or warning signs in the supermarket aisles where there were produce, cleaning products, and insecticides. Nor did I ever see a CAUTION! label next to the entries in the Yellow Pages for pest control services, carpet cleaners, or any of the other countless services dependent on chemicals. In short, I believed that if a product or service was for sale, then it must be safe. However, I am now convinced that this belief may be one of the greatest American myths ever perpetuated.

To see the extent of this myth, we can look at a list of some of the chemicals commonly used for pest control, such as triclopyr (linked to lung cancer), diazinon (linked to various neurotoxic effects), glyphosate (linked to kidney tumors and skin and eye irritations), bendicarb (linked to hyperactivity and vision problems), and chlorpyrifos (linked to neurotoxic effects, including learning disabilities). But such toxic chemicals are not just isolated to pesticides; they can be found almost everywhere.

For example, every year the U.S. produces *nine billion pounds* of formaldehyde, a chemical that has been proven to be carcinogenic in animals. Although not yet proven to cause cancer in humans, formaldehyde can cause such symptoms as headaches, watery eyes, asthma, bronchitis, joint pains, chronic fatigue, disorientation, depression, chest pains, palpitations, chronic ear infections, dizziness, and sinusitis in humans. Yet, despite its toxicity, formaldehyde can be found in a large number of common products, including deodorants, air fresheners, shampoos, mouthwashes, tooth-pastes, cosmetics, orthopedic casts and bandages, facial tissues and napkins, examining table paper rolls, dental bibs, diaper liners, clothing, draperies, carpet, plywood, paint, wallpaper, and more.

According to the California Public Interest Research Group, the U.S. produces a total of *250 billion pounds* of synthetic chemicals each year. Yet, it has been only recently that the media has really begun to present stories about the adverse effects of various chemicals in our lives. In fact, not too long ago, I watched a prime time television special put together by the organization Mothers and Others for a Livable Planet (for which Meryl Streep is the chairperson). As part of the show, Bette Midler entered the stage, full of her usual incredible energy. Smiling and strutting from side to side, she told the audience that she had toned down her act somewhat since she was now a M-O-T-H-E-R. But as she sang and talked about her concerns for this planet, she kept waving her hands with their bright red fingernails. I wanted to shout, "Bette, Bette! Did you know that your nail polish is made from *acetone* and *toluene*, chemicals that can affect the nervous system and possibly cause hearing loss or abnormal liver enlargement?"

But if the Divine Ms. Midler is like most of us, she has probably never thought about the chemical content of her nail polish (or that it has any at all), or how her daughter might be affected by inhaling those chemicals if she sits next to her mother when her nails are being done.

Initially, the realization that toxic chemicals are so intermingled with our daily lives can be very shocking. Part of the reason we may not have previously thought much about our exposures to chemicals is that the conventional medical community has not fully acknowledged the role these chemicals have on our health. Unless a physician is one of those few thousand out of a half million doctors in the United States who has had special training in environmental medicine, he or she probably has little knowledge of the relationship between sickness and the toxins in our environment.

It is not just omissions of warning from the medical profession that helps convince us that everything around us is safe. The scarcity of government regulations restricting or banning toxic chemicals supports the belief that we should not be concerned about the products we use every day. But, history has shown us that just because the government has not regulated a product does not necessarily mean that the product is safe. As long ago as 1914 the dangers of asbestos were so well known that life insurance companies denied policies to individuals who worked with it. However, it was not until almost *sixty years later* that government standards were finally established to protect people from asbestos exposure.

The illusion that everything is safe is further reinforced when manufacturers state that a product has been tested. However, consumers are usually not told that the testing may in fact have been very limited. For example, the majority of products on the market today are rarely tested for any *chronic* adverse health effects. Likewise, testing is often conducted by the manufacturer of the product rather than by independent or government researchers. Many manufacturers commonly finance their own testing since the government does not have the manpower or the budget to do all the testing itself. A prime example of this practice is the cosmetic industry, which assumes total responsibility for all of its testing.

We are also reassured by a product's label which lists all the ingredients in the product. At least that is what we *think* the label tells us. But, in fact, a pesticide manufacturer is only required to list all *active* ingredients. Yet, it is *inert* ingredients that make up most of a product, up to 99 *percent* in some cases. Manufacturers are not required to list the inert ingredients since they are often considered trade secrets. However, many inert ingredients are toxic chemicals and can pose serious health threats. For example, staff members of the EPA have reported that DDT, a chemical banned because of its proven toxicity, is an inert ingredient in several pesticide formulas. Therefore, just because a toxic chemical is not listed on the label does not mean that it is not in the product.

Many people have already been affected by toxic chemicals. According to the U.S. Consumer Product Safety Commission, in 1988 hospital emergency rooms treated more than 2,000 patients for injuries related to household ammonia. (Approximately 40 percent of these cases were children under the age of five.) There were also about 9,000 incidents related to household bleaches (more than 60 percent of theses cases were children under five) and 900 reported cases related to furniture polishes, oven cleaners, and fabric treatment products. (All of these cases involved children under five.) And these statistics represent only *acute* cases; they do not take into account chronic health conditions people experience as a result of daily chemical exposures.

Fortunately, parents *can* do something about reducing their family's exposures to toxins. Parents are not obligated to wait for extensive double-blind studies, specialized laboratory tests, or government policy changes before formulating and acting upon their own personal conclusions. In fact, parents have the power to make *immediate* changes in their family's at any time they choose. They also have the best incentive to do so—the health and well-being of their children.

With that in mind, I wanted to write a book for families. While the information in this book is relevant and applicable to everyone, I have deliberately focused on children. I suspect that some adults may be more receptive to new information if they think something might be adversely affecting *their children*, while they may or may not be motivated to acquire information for themselves.

Throughout each chapter, I rely on my own and my family's experiences, in the hope that they might humanize what may seem like overwhelming information about the potential hazards associated with exposures to chemicals. But just to present our experiences, various statistics, and factual information was not enough for me. I could see no point in writing a book that might shock or scare parents without also providing practical, viable alternatives for change. Therefore, each chapter presents both the problems related to toxic chemicals *and* the solutions and alternatives for reducing the amount of toxic exposures in our lives.

As a wife and mother of two small children, I am greatly motivated to help other families learn this information. If I had known just half of what is presented in this book, my own health and the well-being of my family would be radically different today. I am hoping that upon acquiring this information other families will avoid repeating our mistakes, and, thus, never have to face the hardships we encountered because we blindly believed that just because a product was for sale, it was automatically safe.

Even if some of the chemicals examined in this book are eventually proved to be safe, I do not believe that implementing the alternatives I recommend will be a waste of time. Not only can these suggestions improve our health, but they can also help the planet, which by most accounts is in great jeopardy. On the other hand, if these chemicals are proved to be lethal (as many strongly believe will happen), then these changes will have ensured the health and well-being of many families, as well as preserved a planet for our children.

As a parent, I can afford to believe the very worst—that a product's ingredients are, indeed, toxic—but still give my children the very best (by buying a nontoxic alternative). As I sit here and write, I am trying to think of one thing that had to be eliminated from my two girls' lives since we became committed to reducing the toxins in our lives. But the only thing that I can think of is the countless chemicals confronting them every which way they turned. In our own personal experience, we have been able to find a nontoxic alternative or solution to everything that was previously toxic in our lives.

Making a commitment to seek out alternatives to toxic products remains an individual decision. I, personally, am no longer willing to volunteer my children to participate in the chemical industry's "health effects" test group. (Actually, I've realized I haven't volunteered them at all— I've *paid* for them to participate in this test group by buying product after toxic product.) But I am more than willing to volunteer my family to test nontoxic living each and every day. In fact, I hope that in the near future, nontoxic living will not be considered a challenge or a test, but, rather, an established way of life for everyone.

Quiz 1—A Pretest On Environmental Illness

1. Environmental illness is _____.
> A) a physical health condition resulting from repeated exposures to one or more substances in the environment
> B) a mental health condition resulting from living in crowded, urban areas

2. Environmental illness is often difficult to diagnose because _____.
> A) most doctors trained in traditional medicine have little or no training in environmental medicine
> B) testing for EI is limited, new, and/or controversial
> C) a variety of environmental stimuli may be causing multiple symptoms
> D) all of the above

3. Some people become more chemically sensitive than others because _____.
> A) their immune systems have already been weakened by surgery or chronic illness
> B) they are born with smaller quantities of specific enzymes needed to respond to environmental stimuli
> C) they have already had a greater number of exposures to toxic chemicals
> D) all of the above

4. Adverse reactions to foods and chemicals can cause _____.
> A) mood swings
> B) hyperactivity
> C) poor memory
> D) all of the above

5. New buildings and homes may trigger environmental illness due to _____.
> A) the outgassing of chemicals in building materials
> B) the outgassing of chemicals in new furnishings and finishes
> C) the outgassing of chemicals in new carpets
> D) all of the above

6. According to the National Academy of Sciences, an estimated _____ of the population has some level of chemical sensitivity.
> A) 2 percent
> B) 10 percent
> C) 15 percent
> D) 35 percent

Answers to Environmental Illness Quiz

1. A Environmental illness occurs as the result of an individual's abnormal response to common environmental substances. Environmentally ill persons can have adverse "allergic" reactions that can affect the skin, eyes, ears, nose, throat, lungs, stomach, bladder, vagina, muscles, joints—even the central nervous system, including the brain.

2. D Unfortunately, not only are most doctors unable to recognize environmental illness, but some even deny its existence. Environmental illness can be hard to diagnose because reactions to environmental stimuli can be delayed, sometimes as long as twenty-four hours, and more than one stimulus may be causing a wide variety of symptoms. In these cases, neither the doctor nor the patient can see any clear pattern or relationship between the stimuli and the symptoms.

3. D An already weakened immune system and/or repeated exposures to toxic chemicals can increase the probability of an individual becoming chemically sensitive. However, hereditary factors are usually also involved, since typically more than one family member has some type of allergy. In many cases, an individual had the potential to develop sensitivities but did not begin to experience health problems until the individual's body became overburdened with chemicals.

4. D Mood swings, hyperactivity, poor memory, anxiety, depression, paranoia, and irritability are all common symptoms of chemical reactions.

5. D Many of the chemicals found in new building materials, furnishings, and carpets can cause environmental illness. However, indoor air pollution (as a result of the outgassing of these chemicals) is seldom, if ever, monitored. Indoor air pollution is worst in modern, energy-efficient buildings.

6. C Many people may suffer from chemical sensitivities without even knowing it since they do not associate their symptoms with environmental stimuli. For example, a person who gets a headache whenever he or she goes to a shopping mall might not consider the possibility that he or she is sensitive to formaldehyde and that the headache is a reaction to the excessive amounts of formaldehyde found in malls. However, subtle reactions, such as a headache, should be considered warnings for future potential problems since even minute exposures to chemicals can trigger major adverse reactions once a person has become environmentally ill.

CHAPTER ONE

One Mom's Story

I thought I was a great Mom. I read my children countless stories, encouraged their imaginations, carefully screened babysitters, took them on outings. I even changed professions so I could spend more time at home with them.

I had friends who probably thought they were even better Moms than I: Mothers who breast-fed for an entire year, mothers who would wipe down the shopping cart before putting their children inside it, mothers who never left their babies with anyone other than family members. As Moms, we were each involved in making daily choices that we believed would ensure healthy, wonderful lives for our children.

Then suddenly in January of 1989 I could no longer award myself the title "GREAT MOM." For the first time, I realized that I had been making some daily decisions that had been extremely hazardous to the well-being of my family. At the same time, I also finally realized why I had become so critically ill.

IN THE DARK

In February of 1988 the first sign I had that something was physically wrong with me was that my breasts had started lactating. This would not have been so strange had I not completely stopped breast-feeding my youngest daughter a full ten months earlier. Yet suddenly my breasts were full of milk. About the same time, I noticed that my body had begun to perspire heavily, even though it was winter. This was particularly disturbing since I normally sweated so little that I never needed to use deodorant, even on the hottest summer days. Other than these two peculiar symptoms, I felt fine; but, just to be on the safe side, I set up an appointment with my doctor.

The doctor ordered some blood tests. The results indicated that I "probably" had a pituitary tumor. As the mother of two small children, this was not exactly what I wanted to hear. But, rather than panicking, I got a second opinion. However, the second doctor agreed with the original diagnosis. I spent several subsequent visits to the doctor asking numerous questions before finally agreeing to follow the recommendations of the initial doctor to take medication which would hopefully shrink the tumor.

About a week later, my obstetrician informed me that my class II pap smear indicated the presence of pre-cancerous cells in my cervix and that I would need laser surgery. The doctor assured me the procedure was safe and would eliminate the pre-cancerous cells. I was certainly concerned, but once again, after asking many questions, I agreed to follow the doctor's recommendation.

Confident that everything would be fine, I saw no need to cancel the dinner party planned at my home for the day of the surgery. Nor did I see any need for my husband to accompany me to the doctor's office for the procedure. However, I must confess that once I was lying on the examining table with my legs positioned in the stirrups, I began wishing that maybe I hadn't been so independent.

When I saw the doctor reach for the laser instrument, I suddenly had a desire to have my husband present. The laser instrument reminded me of a blow torch. And I hadn't really internalized that I was going to be just lying there (the nurse gave me a *People* magazine to read) as the doctor literally burned areas of my anesthetized cervix. Feeling somewhat apprehensive, I watched the doctor approach my delicate cervix with the powerful laser in his hand. "Gee, you don't feel the urge to sneeze or anything do you?" I nervously asked.

As I had anticipated, everything went well. I went home, cooked the dinner, entertained my guests, and naturally assumed that everything would be fine. However, three days later, I began experiencing bouts of dizziness and weakness and had a terrible dryness in my mouth. The symptoms would last for a few hours then disappear suddenly. After a few days on this physical roller coaster, I began to suspect the medicine I had been taking for the "alleged" pituitary tumor might be the cause of these symptoms. I called the endocrinologist.

He agreed that it was possible that I was having an allergic reaction to the medicine and suggested that I reduce the dosage. But, when my symptoms still had not abated a few days later, he recommended that I discontinue using the medicine altogether. He would find another type of medication for me and assured me I would start to feel better as soon as the original medication wore off. He was so confident of this that he encouraged me to keep the plans we had made for a weekend family trip, telling me that I would feel much better once I was off the medicine and in the mountains.

Well, his crystal ball must have been on the blink that day, because I spent all of Friday night and all of Saturday in the cabin, unable to get out of bed. To say that I had a "headache" would not do justice to the terrible pain I was experiencing. It felt as if someone were dropping a sixteen pound bowling ball on my head over and over again. Having a headache at all was a new experience for me. In the past, I had always been almost boastful about how aspirin companies would be out of business if they had to depend on customers like me. I believed that weekend I was paying dearly for such testimonials.

Incredibly, by Sunday morning my headache had almost disappeared. I still did not feel completely well, but I felt fit enough to join the family for a hike through the mountains. After breakfast, we headed down the trail. But we didn't get very far before I felt what seemed like small amounts of urine oozing out of me. When I would sit down, it would stop, but as soon as I stood up, it would begin again. Soon after that, I realized that I was hemorrhaging vaginally right there on the mountain trail in the middle of nowhere.

Our first impulse was to quickly return to the cabin, pack up and get to a hospital. However, by the time we returned to the cabin, I was bleeding so much that we realized I needed to go directly to the local fire/paramedic station. Once there, the paramedics immediately hooked me up to an IV and positioned me in the back of their vehicle. The whole event seemed so unreal as I found myself riding down the mountain to the closest hospital some forty miles away.

First Hospital Visit

The doctor in the emergency room examined me and told me that the hemorrhaging was due to a complication from the laser surgery on my cervix. In order to stop the bleeding, he would have to perform surgery. As I had no knowledge of this doctor or hospital, I firmly stated that I wanted to go home to my own doctor (who was about two hours away). But the nice nurse attending me gently said, "Honey, you won't make it home." Judging from all the blood that was still flowing and soaking through the heavy padding on the examining table, I knew she was probably right.

I agreed to have the surgery right then and there. So ended the family retreat to the mountains, but I figured at least the worst was over. The next morning, I was released from the hospital with the doctor's order to stay in bed and rest.

"It"

I had not been home a full day when I began feeling even weaker and sicker than I had been at the hospital. My eyelids swelled up and I was urinating constantly. Then, a few days later, a whole new set of symptoms began to appear—and disappear. For example, one afternoon intense nerve pains suddenly started shooting up and down my left leg; they were so severe that I could not even walk. Another afternoon, while watching Oprah Winfrey, my chest (almost instantly) started burning and a strange racy feeling sped throughout my body.

Very concerned about these latest symptoms, I called the doctor. He said it sounded like an anxiety attack. But that made absolutely no sense to me. Not only had I never previously experienced anything close to an anxiety attack, but I could not imagine what I could be so anxious about in the middle of Oprah Winfrey. (Now, I know that Oprah can be pretty exciting, but not THAT exciting.)

More strange symptoms appeared, but in each case they would disappear as quickly as they had come—only to be replaced by some other strange ailment. I started calling my disease "IT," since I did not now what "IT" was, or when or where "IT" would appear. I kept likening my situation to that of a person continually being poisoned by some evil witch.

As I grew weaker and weaker, the list of symptoms grew longer and longer, and my trips to the doctor became more frequent. When I had first returned from the mountains, my endocrinologist had immediately ordered a brain scan to determine if I did in fact have a pituitary tumor. The results of the brain scan were negative; I had no tumor.

Over the course of the next two weeks, my perplexed endocrinologist referred me to other specialists. In addition to my endocrinologist and obstetrician, whom I saw many times, I saw a gastrologist, a cardiologist, a family practitioner, and a specialist in internal medicine. Each specialist had his or her own diagnosis—Addison's disease, Lupus, Crohn's disease, AIDS, Epstein-Barr, among others. As I would wait for the results of each of these tests, I would ask my husband to get medical books so I could learn more about each proposed disease. But when I read about each one, only a few of my symptoms ever seemed to apply; none of the diseases seemed to really embrace my entire list of symptoms. Even more disturbing was that I usually did *not* have the primary symptom listed as generally associated with the disease. Not surprisingly, after poking and prodding and ordering a battery of tests, none of the doctors could confirm any of these diseases. Moreover, according to blood tests and a variety of diagnostic procedures, I appeared healthy.

But I felt far from healthy. While pondering what course of action to pursue next, a new frightening symptom suddenly appeared one afternoon—I began having difficulty breathing. I kept hoping this symptom would go away as the other symptoms had come and gone. But my breathing only got worse. When I got to the point that I actually could not even talk because I did not have enough oxygen to do so, we called the doctor. He said that I needed to go to the emergency room.

Second Hospital Visit

The emergency room doctor examined me and ordered a number of tests: an EKG, a chest X-ray, and a lung profusion test. The results came back three hours later—negative. According to the tests I was fine. I can still see the doctor standing there telling my husband that there wasn't anything else he could do. He told us to come back if I felt worse.

Still gasping for even a simple breath, I looked at him through puffy, swollen eyelids and could not believe what I was hearing. How could I feel worse? Yet, I was unquestionably being dismissed despite the fact that I was still extremely weak, experiencing a wide variety of symptoms, and having great difficulty breathing.

At home, I found it imperative to make some kind of sense out of what had just happened. I had always believed that when one was critically ill, one went to the emergency room *and got help.* So I rationalized the day's events by convincing myself that I must have had some kind of bad virus. I concluded that the virus had become intensified due to my hemorrhaging, and that somehow this whole weakened condition was affecting my breathing. After all, I reminded myself that even doctors often confess that they really don't know much about viruses.

The next day I *was* worse. But given the previous day's events, I decided not to go back to the emergency room. Actually, I was in such a debilitated state that I was not sure I had the strength to even make it to the car. It was then that my husband and I decided to turn to alternative medicine. Since we knew almost nothing about holistic medicine or doctors who practiced it, we had to rely on the Yellow Pages for a referral.

A Long Three Weeks

As I lay on the bed too weak and breathless to talk, my sister opened the Yellow Pages and turned to the page with the heading ACUPUNCTURE.

She called the first number, but she shook her head as she talked to the person on the other end. "Too weird," she said as she hung up. But during the second call I watched her smile. She told me Dr. Nobu Asano would come to my house to see me. (I must admit that I liked the idea of being treated by a Japanese acupuncturist. It just seemed more authentic.)

Thus began Dr. Asano's regular visits to my home. Every other day he would come and stick numerous needles into my frail body and have me drink a variety of homeopathic teas. During these weeks, I could barely eat and at times I even had trouble sipping water. I was now so weak that my husband had to dress me. To look at me, it seemed incredible that only a few short months ago I was an aggressive tennis player on the court, swam laps in an olympic-sized pool, and coordinated a nationwide basal education program. It did not seem possible that a person's health and life could change so rapidly.

I believed that there was a slight improvement after each acupuncture treatment. But I had no idea how much Dr. Asano was helping me until he had to suddenly go to Japan to visit his ailing mother. Very shortly thereafter, I found it almost impossible to breathe, despite being hooked up to an oxygen tank. For almost every waking minute, I would lie very still in bed and focus on one spot on the wall. As long as I maintained this hypnotic-like trance, I was able to breathe a little easier. But after five days of this incredible mental concentration, I was exhausted. I had used every last bit of my mental energy. Despite trying to believe that I simply had a bad virus, as well as remembering that all the specialists could find nothing wrong with me, I was frightened that my condition had become critical. Unable to speak, I scribbled a note to my mother asking her to call the endocrinologist to see if he would be willing to come to the house.

While one might not believe that a modern-day doctor would ever make a house call, this compassionate doctor did agree to come over. It had been three weeks since I had last seen him, and he later told my husband that it had been very emotional for him to see me in my debilitated state. Only two months earlier, I had walked into his office smiling and making jokes about becoming a wet nurse (via my lactating breasts) as a side profession. But now I was a bedridden, emaciated woman hooked up to oxygen and could barely even whisper to him.

The doctor stressed that I definitely needed to go to the hospital. He assured us that there were other breathing-related tests that the emergency room doctor had not done and that he would personally see that they were ordered for me. Despite my new skepticism of hospitals and specialists, I reluctantly agreed to go. Realistically, I didn't know what other options I had.

Third and Fourth Hospital Visits

After being admitted to the hospital, I met with the pulmonary specialist my endocrinologist had recommended. He didn't inspire much confidence when he told me that as a doctor he himself occasionally had trouble breathing during times of stress. But, in spite of his thinly veiled skepticism, he ordered the tests my doctor wanted.

Later that day, I underwent a grueling pulmonary function test. When the results indicated asthma, an excited technician went to find the pulmonary specialist. The partner of the pulmonary specialist was now on duty, and he confirmed that I did have asthma. As strange as it may seem, we were all ecstatic—finally and explanation for why I couldn't breathe, a name for my condition, a condition that could be treated!

The doctor prescribed asthma medication which I began immediately. The medication was a significant stimulant for me since I was not even accustomed to drinking coffee. After one month of not being able to talk because I did not have enough air to breathe *and* converse, you could not shut me up. Not only was I excited to have finally been diagnosed, but I was also happy and enthusiastic about going home.

The happiness and enthusiasm, however, were short-lived. Less than twenty-four hours later, I had trouble breathing again. At first I thought I was not taking a strong enough dosage of the asthma medication, as it had been explained to me that dosages varied among patients. My husband and I called the medical clinic but could not get either pulmonary specialist to return our calls. After a phone conversation with my endocrinologist, we discovered that the two pulmonary doctors disagreed about my diagnosis. (The original pulmonary specialist was not convinced that I had asthma.) The specialist who had diagnosed the asthma and had put me on the medication was now backing off the case since technically I was not his patient. It was confusing and frustrating. But worst of all, I was having even more difficultly breathing. We called the first pulmonary specialist once more, and he finally returned our call at 8:00 P.M. that night. He said that I should go to the emergency room if I felt it were necessary. By midnight, we decided we had no other option.

This was the same emergency room I had visited the first time I could not breathe three weeks earlier. But this time it was different. All I had to say was that I had been diagnosed two days ago as having asthma, and the next thing I knew the doctors had pumped me with so much adrenaline that my pulse shot up to over 150 and my body could not stop shaking. I remember thinking that this "cure" was about as bad as not being able to breathe.

Five hours later, I returned home, weary and still not feeling like I was breathing well, though I was doing better.

That morning we made an appointment with the original pulmonary specialist to see about changing my medication, which the emergency room doctor had recommended. I thought there would now be no doubt in the specialist's mind about my asthma condition since a whole emergency room team had treated me for an intensive asthma attack just eight hours earlier.

He agreed to see me, but the first thing he did when I was in his office was to give me another kind of asthma test using a different machine. He did not share the results of the test, but he assured me that I would not have asthma for very long. He did not believe it necessary to change the dosage of asthma medication that his partner had prescribed.

But, less than twenty-four hours later, I was once again having great difficulty breathing. Neither pulmonary specialist would return my call. It was like a recurring nightmare. I was determined to avoid another emergency room visit as I feared that my body could not endure any more adrenaline. Not knowing what else to do, I called my family doctor whom I had not seen since I had hemorrhaged. He examined me and confirmed that I was having an asthma attack. He told me I needed to go on steroids for a short period of time in order to breathe properly. I loathed the thought of being on steroids, but I was desperate and believed him. More than anything, I just wanted to be able to breathe effortlessly.

When I took my first dose of steroids, it was time, once again, to have our home sprayed by our bi-monthly pest control service for our never-ending problem with fleas. Despite the fact that all the doctors I had seen thus far had reassured me that the pesticides could not be affecting my breathing, I wanted to be out of the house the night after the service came to spray. Considering my two recent asthma attacks, I just didn't want to take any chances. We made reservations to spend the night in a nearby hotel.

But that one night turned into six nights of the closest thing to hell I think I'll ever know. Almost as soon as I started taking the steroids, I began experiencing a series of symptoms that racked my body and my spirit. My chest was burning so badly that it felt as if someone had pressed hot coals into it. And, I suddenly became so sensitive to noise and stimuli that I couldn't even watch TV. Unbelievably, I also did not even want to be around my very own children. For the first time during this whole ordeal, I wasn't sure that I wanted to live any longer.

I refused to leave the hotel room. Due to the combined stimulant effect of the steroids and the asthma medications, I had probably slept a total of eight hours over the past five days—and that was only with the help of sleeping pills, something I had never taken before. I was tense, speedy and withdrawn. It was as if a completely different person was masquerading in my body. On top of all this, I still was not breathing normally, although there had been some improvement. It was in the middle of this horrible time that I received a report from the original pulmonary specialist which nearly sent me over the edge: there was NO EVIDENCE that I had asthma.

But if this was true, then WHY had he kept me on all these horrible medications—even after I told him they were too strong for me. Why had the entire ER team shot me with adrenaline? What had my family doctor heard when he had listened to my chest and then insisted that I needed steroids? And, if I didn't have asthma, then WHY was I even on these terrible steroids? I was nearly hysterical.

Now there was a new diagnosis for me—mental illness. Up until this time (with the exception of the first pulmonary specialist), the doctors I had seen had always treated me as if they believed there *was* something physically wrong with me—they just did not know what. I had no prior history of being a person who went from doctor to doctor. I was always calm and logical during doctor visits, and I had absolutely no reason to "fake" an illness to escape from the world.

But now, after all the referrals since my hemorrhaging, one could make a case that I *was* a person who went from doctor to doctor complaining of a long list of symptoms. In the hotel room, I *was* irrational. I absolutely refused to go home if there was even the slightest smell of pesticides; I ranted and raved about how the pulmonary specialist had deceived me; and I insisted that no more than one person at a time be in the hotel room with me.

Not surprisingly, the latest doctor's recommendation was to institutionalize me. My family even temporarily considered this; they were mentally and physically drained, very confused, and could no longer offer an explanation for my sudden, dramatic change in behavior.

To tell the truth, I might have even accepted being classified as crazy, as long as the others acknowledged that it was possible to be insane *and* have a real physical ailment. But I was afraid that if they "locked me away" I would never discover the source of my symptoms, which I was convinced were physical in origin. I believed this because while I had lost twenty pounds and a lot of blood from the vaginal hemorrhaging, I was *still* lactating! When I used to breast-feed my daughters, my milk supply would be greatly reduced if I had even the slightest cold or became run down. Therefore, I found it incredible that as weakened as I had become, I was still producing breast milk. I knew that I could not prove that I wasn't imagining my breathing difficulties, my burning chest, or that racy sensation which overwhelmed my body at times. But the doctors and my family could not deny that the milk filling my breasts was real, and, thus far, medical science had no explanation for it. So I pleaded with my family to not consider institutionalizing me at least until I was off the steroids.

As they listened to my request, they agreed that my dramatic behavior changes had begun almost immediately after taking the steroids. And, unlike the latest doctor, my family had known me for years. With confidence, they knew that I had never been a whining, hysterical woman, wanting to hide from the world. Instead, they knew me as a person who was typically characterized as decisive, confident, and creative—sometimes feisty and stubborn—but never, never as nuts.

They agreed to wait. As I had hoped, when the drugs passed out of my system, my erratic behavior disappeared. I was no longer hysterical; I could handle noise; and I wanted to see and hug my children. Most of all, I wanted to go home.

Yet, after just a few hours in my home, I was having difficulty breathing again. I feared I was beginning to sound like a broken record. We were back to square one—in search of a new doctor.

Doctor of the Week

By now, I had seen so many doctors that I had begun thinking of them in terms of numbers instead of names. Doctor 16 gave me the established "challenge test" to determine once and for all if I had asthma. The test came back negative, and he took me off all the original asthma medications. While I was relieved to be off the medicine, I was still in the dark as to what was really wrong with me. I wanted to know *why* I was having difficulty breathing, *why* I was lactating, *why* I could barely even stand up, and *why* I had no appetite. Doctor 16 had no answers for these questions; he could only tell me that I did not have asthma.

Doctor 17 had an answer: a sinus X-ray showed that I had a sinus infection. He proposed that the infection had dripped down into my lungs as a result of laying in bed, day after day, weakened from the hemorrhaging. He explained that this, in turn, had affected my bronchial tubes, which then impaired my breathing. It seemed plausible, and we were again relieved to finally know the cause of my physical problems and to have a name for my mystery condition. I eagerly started the antibiotics he prescribed.

But after six weeks and three rounds of antibiotics, my condition had still not improved. The doctor then told me I needed sinus surgery to remove the infection. Cautious because of my recent experiences with the medical community, I took the X-rays to FOUR other doctors for additional opinions. Three unquestionably agreed that I needed the surgery. Only one doctor told me not to have the surgery—my acupuncturist who had returned from Japan. He did not claim to know the cause of my illness, but he insisted that from the perspective of Eastern medicine, my sinuses were *not* the source of my problem. He was concerned that such a major operation would severely stress my already over-drugged, exhausted body. I was concerned about his comments, but desperately wanted to breathe normally. At that point, I probably would have done just about anything if I thought it would have helped me breathe better. So, in the end, I opted for the operation.

Fifth Hospital Visit

I knew something was wrong the minute the general anesthesia from the operation wore off and I came to. I was extremely weak—which I had expected—but I also experienced that racy feeling I had had at other times since my laser surgery. It felt as if the inside of my body was the roadway at the Indianapolis 500, and cars were zooming around at breakneck speeds. I was too weak to stand, too hyper to lie down. In the hospital bed, I would turn to the left, to the right, and back to the left. All I kept thinking was that I wanted to crawl out of my skin.

The nurse thought I might be having a negative reaction to the anesthesia that would pass as soon as it wore off. Unfortunately, I remained this way for almost two days. On the third day, I was released from the hospital with the doctor's glowing report. In his eyes, my recovery was going well, and he was optimistic about the success of the surgery.

Home Again

I certainly wanted to believe him. Yet, within a couple of days, any optimistic thoughts about the sinus surgery were gone—not that anyone around me wanted to hear that. "Give it time," they all said. But I knew better. I knew what I was feeling, and I was definitely in worse condition than I had been before the surgery. For example, one evening I suddenly became so weak that it felt like every system in my body had just shut down. I remember fighting hard to stay conscious, remaining in a half-alive condition for more than two hours. On a regular basis, my throat now felt so tight that I imagined that a boa constrictor was around my neck, wrapping itself tighter and tighter.

At the post-operative office visit, I told the doctor that I believed the sinus surgery had *not* helped me and that I feared something else was still very wrong. But he did not want to hear that. I remember him curtly saying,

"You're just going to have to accept that it is the 1980s and no one knows what's wrong with you!" Looking back, I'm sure his words were prompted by his own frustration. But, at the time, I thought, "Well, maybe *he* can accept that it's the 1980s and that *he* doesn't know what's wrong with me. But, I can't accept that." I was determined to discover the true source of my symptoms.

Needless to say, I went to a new physician, Doctor 21, who ended up sending me to Doctor 22. Doctor 22 ran some tests to determine why my throat felt so tight. However, the results did not really provide any new insights. Nevertheless, he prescribed some medicine to relax the muscles in my throat, even though he had no idea what was causing it to happen if, in fact, he even really believed it *was* happening. But immediately after taking the medicine, I once again got that horrible racy sensation. As much as I wanted relief for my throat, this "crawling out of my skin" sensation was too high a price to pay.

Since I could not seem to tolerate the medicine he first prescribed, the doctor then prescribed a heart medication, a beta blocker, even though I did not have a heart condition. He explained that a side effect of beta blockers was that they relaxed muscles. It seemed very strange to prescribe a heart medication for me. But, although I was confused, I asked my father to fill the prescription, as he had all the others.

When my father returned from the pharmacy, I was lying on the couch, unable to talk since the "boa constrictor" was around my throat. Sensing my urgency, my father handed me the new heart (but for me, throat) medication. But, instead of opening it, I just looked at the bottle for a very long time. The desire to rid myself of the "boa constrictor" around my throat was overwhelming, but there was something else more powerful within me that kept me from taking those pills. I then made a decision that I now realize was a significant turning point. I handed the bottle back to my Dad.

For the first time, my situation became very clear to me. My kitchen cupboards were so full of prescription drugs from twenty-two doctors that I probably could have opened my own pharmacy. But in truth, none of these drugs had helped, and most had produced some negative side effects in me. I did not want to take drugs that *might* help, and I did not want to rely on drugs for the rest of my life. I wanted to know WHY my throat felt like it was closing up, WHY after thirty-three years I was having trouble breathing, and WHY I was too weak to even stand up. Therefore, I decided to stop all the medications until I knew the answers to these questions. While I continued to search, I would only consent to acupuncture and herbal teas.

My resolve weakened when after one month I was no better. I was so discouraged that I finally agreed to see the last doctor to whom I had been referred (since I was told that he could run some tests that, amazingly, I had not yet taken). When those tests also came back normal, I wasn't really surprised when he began making a strong pitch for anti-depressant drugs. According to his diagnosis, I had been a strong, healthy, independent woman who had suffered a series of very unfortunate misdiagnoses but who now had nothing physically wrong with her. He thought I was having a hard time accepting that. He looked me straight in the eye and sincerely told me that if I took the anti-depressant drugs, he thought I would be back to my former healthy condition *within a month.*

I know he believed what he was saying, and the idea of ending this nightmare in one month sounded absolutely wonderful. I had been completely incapacitated for five months now and wanted more than anything to be a functioning wife, mother, and writer again. But something inside me knew that anti-depressant drugs were not the answer—no matter how much the doctor told me they would help me and "couldn't hurt me." To his dismay, I told him not to even bother to write the prescription.

My visits with Doctor 23 had not been a complete waste of time, however. During my consultation with him, he had revealed the contents of the surgeon's report on my sinus surgery. It seems as though what the surgeon had removed was a sinus infection I had had for over *twenty* years, and, therefore, it could not have been the cause of my recent problems. Doctor 23 added that the surgeon must have known that there was little chance that he was going to find a new infection since there had been no indication of one during a pre-surgery procedure the week before.

I didn't even react. While I had certainly felt angry at times with Doctors 14 through 22, now I was just numb. I figured that if there was such a thing as reincarnation, then I must have done something pretty awful in my previous life. So, despite five hospital visits, twenty-three different doctors, and a possible world record for ingesting the most medications within a five-month period, I was still completely incapacitated. My current symptoms were extreme weakness, dizziness, throat swelling, shortness of breath, diarrhea, nerve burning and numbness, chest pain, and more.

The Candida Connection

During this entire time, I continued to have acupuncture as I believed the treatments were relieving some of my symptoms. One day Dr. Asano mentioned something about a condition called Candida. He explained that when the immune system was impaired (as no doubt mine was), an overgrowth of Candida albicans (yeast) could result. He added that some doctors were now convinced that this overgrowth could then trigger a chronic health condition producing a variety of symptoms similar to what I was experiencing.

I immediately sent my sister out to find a book on the subject. She came back with the only book on Candida she could find. I eagerly began to read. I quickly became very excited. It was like the author had known me! Even some of my strangest symptoms were right there in print! But what really struck me was that the author, a doctor, claimed that Candida often gained a foothold in the bodies of persons who had taken numerous antibiotics. When I thought about how many antibiotics I had taken orally and intravenously in the last five months, I was convinced that Candida was somehow connected to my ill-health.

The next problem, however, was trying to locate a doctor who believed Candida overgrowth could cause multiple, chronic health problems. Most doctors only believe that yeast can cause a little vaginal discomfort (commonly referred to as a "yeast infection") or oral thrush. They do not believe that Candida overgrowth can cause something which could be systemic and affect the entire body. However, it did not bother me that systemic Candida was being debated in the conventional medical community since, thus far, my experiences with that group had not improved my health. Moreover, the treatment for this chronic health condition seemed so harmless—especially when compared to laser surgery, sinus surgery, steroids, or any of the other procedures and medications that had been prescribed for me.

The medical doctor I found a few weeks later put me on a yeast-free and sugar-free diet and gave me nutritional supplements and an anti-fungal tea. Within a month, I noticed a marked improvement. Specifically, I was not nearly as weak. Yet, I still had many symptoms. There was still something very wrong.

THE GREAT DISCOVERY

While I improved with the Candida treatment, I grew concerned over new symptoms which seemed to be neurological in origin. Often sharp nerve pains shot up and down the left side of my body, and I was continually dizzy. By now, I had read three more books on Candida and had become convinced that I might also be suffering from a specific endocrine condition noted as common to people with systemic Candida. There was a specific test to determine whether or not one had this condition, so I contacted one of the doctors listed in the books and set up an appointment.

When I entered this doctor's office, I noticed a number of signs referring to "detox patients." I had no idea what these signs meant. The doctor's questions were similarly peculiar. How many times had we sprayed our house with pesticides? How old was my home? Did the floors have new carpet? This questioning went on for about forty minutes until finally the doctor simply announced that he believed I was being poisoned *by my very own home.*

By this time, I had probably received more than two dozen diagnoses, but this one, strange as it sounded, instinctively seemed right. It was the first diagnosis that corresponded with the sequence of events and the symptoms which had followed. There in the doctor's office, I immediately remembered how I had returned from the mountains following my second cervix surgery. I recalled that our house had just been sprayed by our bi-monthly pest control service and that a strong pesticide odor had lingered longer than usual—three weeks, in fact. And while the rest of my family had gone in and out of the house, I had stayed inside the entire time while I recovered from the surgery. It was during this time that I first began having trouble breathing.

Suddenly, all my bizarre reactions to the countless medications also made sense as the doctor continued to explain. My severe reactions were due to the fact that my body had become so toxic that it could not handle any other drugs in my system. The chest burning in the hotel room was not my imagination but the result of adding more chemicals—steroids, asthma medications, sleeping pills—to my toxic body every four hours, thus triggering nonstop physical and mental allergic-like reactions.

As I sat there it also became obvious why I had felt *worse* after my sinus surgery. I remembered that I had come home to recuperate in a house that had, once again, been sprayed with pesticides. It now became clear to me why every time I returned home I experienced difficulty breathing. In short, I was being poisoned by the pesticides and other chemicals, primarily formaldehyde, that were outgassing from the furniture, carpet and construction materials of my new home.

In retrospect, I could see that for the two-and-a-half years we had lived in our new home my body had been storing pesticides and other toxic chemicals. My detoxification system was most likely already overloaded when I began taking the medication for the pituitary tumor. The anesthesia and stress from my first two surgeries, combined with trying to recuperate in a home continually sprayed with pesticides, undoubtedly expedited my rapid downward spiral to ill-health.

The doctor, trained in environmental medicine, further explained that this on-going chemical poisoning had been impairing my entire immune system. He wanted to order some special blood tests which he believed would confirm high levels of chemical toxicity in my body. I agreed to the tests, but I decided not to wait for the results before entering the detox program he offered for patients. My instincts told me this therapy was going to help. Until now, I had allowed others in authoritative positions to persuade me that there was no basis for my instincts. Yet, I could not help but recall that all along I had intuitively believed that the pesticide smell *had* affected me. I had only stopped being persistent on this point after so many doctors told me it was not possible. Therefore, I didn't want to wait to see if my insurance was going to cover the costs of the program. Nor was I influenced by the fact that I was told it was a very controversial program. I didn't care. I wanted to get well, and I firmly believed that the road to recovery started at the detox clinic.

THE DETOX CLINIC

I decided to enter the detox program the very next day. The actual detox area consisted of a large room in a back wing of a medical facility. In the room were five saunas, each of which had been constructed out of a different type of wood in order to accommodate the chemical sensitivities of the patients. It was explained that some patients were so sensitive to certain materials that they could not tolerate being next to or sitting on certain types of woods. I thought this a little extreme, only to later discover that I could not tolerate the sauna made from cedar. Next to each sauna was a large white chair.

In the center of the room was the nurse's desk, which faced the exercise equipment (exercise bikes and a small trampoline) the patients used to get their circulation moving when they first arrived. The only other piece of furniture in the room was a massage-type table which was pushed against one of the walls. This nondescript table, as I would soon find out, played an important role in the detox program.

The nurse explained the treatment I would be undergoing. I would be given nutrient supplements and daily doses of niacin to help release the toxins from the fatty tissues where they are stored. In addition, I would undergo physical therapy. But the main part of the treatment would center around the saunas in which I would be required to sit for three hours a day. Set at 180 degrees, the saunas would cause me to literally sweat out the toxins that had accumulated in my tissues and had been released into my bloodstream by the other therapies and treatments of the program. I would undergo six thirty-minute sessions every day, including weekends, for three to six weeks, depending on how well I was progressing.

I thought it all sounded fine. After all, I joked with the nurse, if sweat baths were good enough for our Native Americans, then surely a little perspiring couldn't hurt me. However, I seemed to overlook one major factor— Native Americans were not sweating out pesticides, formaldehyde, toluene. . . .

On my first day at the clinic, I discovered why the chairs were next to each sauna. At times, I would watch patients come out of a sauna feeling too weak or sick to move. They would just sink into the closest chair. But then there were times when the chairs were just not enough. I was alarmed on those first few days as I watched some patients get carried to the massage table against the wall.

Typically, the nurse would then rush over with the blood pressure equipment and/or oxygen. The doctor would usually appear moments later. I would only watch from a distance, but it seemed that whomever was on the table either was crying or was too weak to even make a sound.

Then, I could hardly believe it when I would watch the staff make the patient leave the table and GET BACK INTO THE SAUNA to finish sweating out rest of the toxins that had been stirred up and had been coming out too quickly. I used to think that those patients had true courage to return to the sauna. I never dreamed that *I* would ever end up on the table facing the same challenge.

As I sat in the saunas each day, I began to get to know some of the other patients. Most had flown in from other parts of the country. All were hoping to detox the chemicals that had been impairing their health. These patients told of intolerances to chemical smells, countless doctors who had given incorrect diagnoses, a history of taking antibiotics, and futile emergency room visits which had left them in worse shape. The duplication of symptoms and experiences among people who had never previously conversed was absolutely incredible to me.

I became friends with many of the patients: Mary,* whose neurological symptoms and ill-health were the direct result of an overdose spraying by their monthly pest control company; Laura, who always seemed to be in a "fog" from years of breathing toxic solvents at her job in a printing plant; Liz, who had become critically ill from living near a toxic waste dump. There were also children: Paul, who had had life-threatening asthma from the time he was a toddler as a result of the chemicals used in the construction of his mobile home; Joseph, in whom the solvent-based adhesives used for his braces had triggered a neurological condition which caused his eyes to pull back to one side and then into his head; Susan and Kyle, who had un-

* Some names throughout the book have been changed.

predictable seizures caused by the confirmed high concentration of formaldehyde in their new home.

Then I met Bill and Shelly. Bill was the head of a state department in Kentucky and Shelly was his executive secretary. Both (as well as twenty others who remained in Kentucky) had become chronically ill from working in a "sick building." Before I met Bill and Shelly, all I kept thinking was that the detox clinic was going to be a very depressing environment in which to spend the next six weeks. I had decided that I would try to make the hours pass with as much levity as possible. With Bill and Shelly, this became possible.

First, Bill would keep us laughing with his on-going commentary about Californians from his native Kentuckian perspective. I remember one day when he entered the clinic loudly exclaiming in his distinct Southern drawl, "I can't believe it! You all have hotels out here that rent *by the hour*!!" On other days, Bill, Shelly and I would resort to singing bluegrass songs as we tried to pass what seemed like the endless time inside our sauna. When we witnessed weird events, such as a patient detoxing small white crystals out of her skin that caused the dyes of her bathing suit to run together, we would start humming the theme song to *The Twilight Zone*. As the writer of the group, I nicknamed the place "As the Chemicals Turn" and created daily soap opera episodes about the lives of the patients. To make things more interesting and juicy, I would often throw in some wild fabrications about some of the staff. Whenever possible, we would laugh. We laughed so much that our sauna came to be known as the "fun sauna."

We searched for humor because the alternative was to sit in those saunas and dwell on the fears that each of us were silently experiencing: the fear of when the next layer of toxins would dump into our bloodstream, the fear of whether or not the detox program was really helping, and the fear of how we were going to ever survive in such a chemical world. But despite our efforts to bring some levity to the place, there were some days when the chemicals we were detoxing were so powerful that laughter was just not possible.

When I first began detoxing, almost immediately my face and hands started turning different shades of yellow and orange—not just tints of these colors but bright, unmistakable shades of yellow and orange. Along with my new coloring, I experienced continual nausea and a variety of neurological symptoms. Then, just as I was getting used to my new tie-dyed look, blurry vision, and sea-sickness-on-land, my symptoms began to change.

On the fourteenth day of detox, I started experiencing allergic symptoms, such as eyelid swelling, while I was in the sauna! I kept thinking,

"What can I be allergic to in a sauna???" As incredible as it seemed, I soon discovered that I was reacting to a layer of pesticide toxins emitting from my body! I was actually beginning to reek of the pesticides that had been sprayed in my home. With each subsequent sauna that day, I smelled even worse. Several of the patients at the clinic who were sensitive to pesticides had to stay away from me as I triggered adverse reactions in them.

The same smell persisted the following day. After my third sauna, I plopped down on one of the white chairs. Then, all of the sudden, my body went into a tailspin. My heart and chest started burning, my blood pressure dropped, and suddenly it seemed as if someone had swept the floor out from under me. I tried to stand but my legs (what I could barely feel of them) felt like jello. I think the nurse understood what was happening before I did as she jumped up from behind the desk. I knew where I was going—to the dreaded table next to the wall.

For two hours I lay on that table, shivering and scared as toxins overwhelmed my body. Anne, another patient at the clinic whom I had nicknamed "The Champ" because she was on her seventy-third day of detox, stood beside me. Two and a half months earlier, Anne had entered the clinic in a wheelchair, hooked up to oxygen, and barely alive. Now she was off almost all her medication and was driving herself to the clinic each day. She, more than anyone, knew how it felt when the toxins in your body suddenly dumped into your bloodstream. I remember her telling me, "You survived the pesticides going in the first time, and you'll survive them going out. You will." Fortunately, she was right.

My sessions continued, but the following week was not much easier. Every day I spent a total of three hours sweating out toxins in the sauna. I was now sweating so much that I was drinking approximately 180 ounces of water a day to replace the fluids I was losing.

On my twenty-third day of detox, I decided to quit. I knew that I had not yet nearly detoxed all the chemicals stored in me, but my body and spirit could no longer stand the stress. I hoped that I had sweated out enough chemicals so that my liver could once again function properly. I hoped that my body would continue to rid itself of the residual chemicals naturally.

LIVING IN A TOXIC WORLD

Even after leaving the detox clinic, I really had not accepted that I was a person who reacted to a long list of everyday chemicals. It still seems incredible to me that only a short time ago I was a person with *no* allergies. Yet today I have what is referred to as environmental illness, or multiple chemical sensitivities. What happened to me and to most others with this health condition is that an initial overexposure to certain chemicals, in my case primarily pesticides and formaldehyde, had triggered sensitivities to another long, long list of other everyday chemicals.

Almost overnight, I was faced with living and functioning in a world to which I was allergic. Suddenly, it seemed as if paints, fertilizers, and household cleaners were everywhere. In the short time I was at the clinic, it seemed as if the nurseries in my neighborhood had multiplied, and I was convinced that the pest control companies were sending convoys of their trucks just to circle my home. I could no longer enter a department, toy, or grocery store because the various products on the shelves outgassed a wide variety of chemicals that adversely affected me. I could not go to the movies as the perfumes and scents of the other patrons would also trigger reactions. I could not fill up my car with gas because the fumes would almost knock me unconscious. It seemed as if everything had changed. Yet I knew that really the only thing that had changed was my perception of the world. I now saw an unsafe world that most perceived as harmless.

I readily acknowledge that many people do not believe that daily chemicals can harm us. Their perceived good health is their proof, and the present controversy over environmental illness within the medical community only reinforces such beliefs. But, personally, I cannot share this viewpoint. Prior to my illness, I was just the average mother, wife, and professional; there was no warning or indication that I would soon become proof that common, everyday chemicals can make us ill. Now when I hear "authorities" discredit any hazards associated with daily chemicals by claiming that the level of exposure is "too minute to cause any harm," I know better. I did not live in Love Canal or next to the pesticide plant that blew up in India, nor did I work with toxic chemicals. I was only exposed to those same "too minute to cause any harm" levels that so many continue to insist are safe.

Yet, as I continue to live nontoxically and to detox naturally, I do note improvement. In fact, some of my sensitivities have already decreased significantly. Not too long ago, I had to actually "bake" any new book, magazine, or newspaper before reading it as the fresh print produced reactions. ("Hey, has anyone seen the *Time* magazine?" "Sure, just look in the oven.") Fortunately, this is no longer necessary. It is these kinds of improvements that encourage me to believe that slowly, very slowly, I may also become less sensitive to many other chemicals. But when people repeatedly ask me, "Do you think you will ever get back to the way you were before?" I do not have the answer.

MAKING THE CHANGES

When I left the clinic I knew that my lifestyle and that of my family was going to have to change dramatically. But, I must confess, my first thought was, "Oh, no! my days of being blonde and permed are over." Clearly, this was not to be the most significant area of change, but I suppose that I was really afraid to face just how different our lives were going to have to be. Yet, since I was determined to get well, I was willing to make whatever changes were necessary. The first obvious thing we did was cancel the pest control service. About the same time, we began buying organic fruits and vegetables as well as meats that did not contain any growth hormones or antibiotics. Next, we threw away all our chemical cleaning products and replaced them with natural alternatives. Last, we sold our home.

Our real estate agent had the great challenge of finding us a house that had never been sprayed with pesticides and was not downwind from a nursery or toxic dump. Our next residence could also not be a new home, since all the outgassing chemicals from the construction materials would trigger reactions in me, and it could not be an old home with multiple past owners as we had to be able to trace the pesticide record of the home. Finding this home in southern California was not going to be easy.

A month later we bought a two-year-old house from the original owners who signed a sworn statement saying that they had never used or employed others to spray pesticides in the home. But once we bought the house, the real work was just beginning. We had only one week prior to moving in to make all the necessary changes.

With a lot of careful coordinating, however, everything was completed on schedule. All the carpeting was ripped out and replaced with tiles and hardwood floors that had been laid without glues and had been sealed with a nontoxic finish. The pressed wood cabinets were sealed with a nontoxic sealant to keep them from outgassing formaldehyde. The garage, which shared a common wall with the kitchen, was sealed off with an aluminum vapor barrier, keeping gas fumes out of the house. We had a house-wide water purifying system installed and replaced the gas-fed range and water heater with electric ones. Last of all, we bought a sauna so I could continue my daily detox sessions at home.

Every time we learned something new about toxic effects, we looked for alternatives and solutions. We had hoped to see long-term results, but we were surprised with the immediate changes. Within weeks of moving into our new home, the undiagnosed skin rash on both my girls' faces disappeared. Winter arrived, but the usual runny noses and colds did not. At the same time, my husband, a part-time triathlete, began noticing that he was training harder, while sleeping less, and breaking personal records at races. And, without question, I was making the continual health improvements that we had hoped for when we moved.

IN THE FUTURE

I sincerely hope that government policy and the mainstream medical society will begin to seriously acknowledge the cause and effect relationship between chemicals and health. But, in the interim, I am grateful that both resources and options are available for those choosing to living nontoxic lifestyles.

To the surprise of many, I actually prefer my new lifestyle, even though (thus far) it is still complicated by many, many health problems. In some very real ways, I am actually grateful for everything that has happened—even though this statement usually stuns most people who expect legal action and anger to be more appropriate reactions. But these persons would have no way of knowing how much I have come to value the information I have acquired as a result of becoming ill.

I do not believe that anyone ever tried to maliciously hurt me or act in any way other than what they thought to be appropriate at the time. Moreover, no one forced me to employ a pesticide service or consent to numerous surgeries. In the end, I ultimately made each of those decisions, and, therefore, I take full responsibility for all the consequences that followed. For me, this perspective is a key part of my healing as it clearly reminds me that I am also the person responsible for regaining my strength and health.

While I accept the responsibility for my actions and do not blame others, I also do not blame myself for the past harmful decisions I made for my family. Instead, I have chosen to believe that all the characters in my story, including myself, simply shared a lack of knowledge. It is this knowledge that I am now motivated to bring to as many people as possible. It is this knowledge that enables me to no longer feel vulnerable or helpless in a world full of chemicals.

But I do not deny that part of my challenge is to try and educate as many people who are willing to learn. Environmental illness is one of the most preventable diseases around—once one knows about it and believes in its existence. Therefore, I share my story not only to humanize the impact of these toxic chemicals in our lives but to encourage people to acquire this knowledge for themselves. By doing so, hopefully, others can become enlightened without experiencing part or all of what happened to me. I especially hope that children will benefit from this information not only because I am a mother but because, one-and-a-half years later, I still cannot shake the image of those children at the detox clinic. They were there simply because their parents (like most of us) had no idea that toxic chemicals were in their children's lives.

I readily concede that it is disturbing and frightening to believe that our lives may be filled with harmful chemicals. But I am hoping that parents will not reject acquiring information simply because they find it threatening or unbelievable. Instead, I am hoping that parents will find it more frightening and threatening to remain uninformed. Likewise, acquiring knowledge of nontoxic alternatives and products is not synonymous with a commitment to make changes. That remains the choice of each individual. My hope in presenting both my story and the information that follows is to bring an awareness to parents so that they can truly feel they are making educated choices for their children.

At times, I confess I am overwhelmed by the challenge of sharing this information. I sometimes forget that others have not yet had an opportunity to be exposed to these facts or have not experienced the adverse effects of these chemicals firsthand. Forgetting this, I sometimes get taken aback when I hear that someone who does not know me has responded to my story by saying something like, "Does this woman have all her marbles? She's not some kind of nut is she?" This kind of comment disturbs me not because it places a doubt on what I have come to know as fact but because it reminds me of how little information so many people presently have.

But I am optimistic, simply because it was not that long ago that I might have made such a comment. I do not forget that my life and my family's environment had just as many chemicals in it as the next person's—maybe even more. Yet, I am now proof that a nontoxic lifestyle can be both possible and appreciated even by a self-proclaimed "yuppie" like myself. I am encouraged when I hear my friends report significant improvement in their own children's health after reducing exposures to daily chemicals. Last of all, I remain hopeful because I truly believe that when parents do acquire the overwhelming information about the chemicals in our environment, they simply will no longer be willing to gamble with their sons' and daughters' lives.

CHECKLIST FOR SUGGESTED CHANGES
AND COMMITMENTS

☐ Begin reading up on health, environmental illness and related issues. Also begin reading books offering nontoxic alternatives. See Appendix 1 for a list of suggested readings.

☐ Join the Human Ecology Action League (HEAL), an organization dedicated to minimizing or eliminating pesticides and toxic chemicals in our lives. Members receive the quarterly publication *The Human Ecologist* which provides updated information on environmental health issues and suggestions for nontoxic alternatives. See Appendix 2 for address.

☐ Challenge the generally accepted notion that we should *expect* to catch five to six "colds" a year, experience a winter-long runny nose, suffer through repeated ear infections, and so forth. If you are experiencing repeated illnesses, consult a doctor trained in environmental medicine to find out if food and/or chemicals are contributing to or triggering your symptoms. Consult the American Academy of Environmental Medicine (address in Appendix 2) to locate practicing physicians in your area.

Quiz 2—A Pretest on Pesticides

1. Claims that pesticides are safe "when used as directed" are

_____.

      A) illegal

      B) legal

2. Children who live in homes in which household and garden pesticides are used have a _____ greater chance of developing childhood leukemia.[1]

      A) two times

      B) four times

      C) seven times

3. In a 1983 San Francisco survey, _____ was found to be the most common pesticide residue found on fresh produce.[2]

      A) malathion

      B) DDT

      C) Round-up

4. Since the use of agricultural pesticides has increased tenfold in the last thirty years, crop losses due to insects have _____.

      A) been halved

      B) doubled

      C) tripled

5. A pesticide that has been previously banned for use in this country can still be used if _____.

      A) the EPA grants an emergency waiver

      B) the manufacturer submits new testing

6. Banned pesticides can still be manufactured in this country as long as

_____.

      A) companies provide on-going health and safety data

      B) the pesticides are intended for export

      C) they are not transported anywhere

7. In a survey of 900 homes that use a pest control service, _____ of the homes showed pesticide levels higher than expected for correct applications.

      A) 10 percent

      B) 25 percent

      C) 64 percent

8. Of the approximate 50,000 home pesticide poisonings each year, _____ are children under the age of four.

      A) 5,000

      B) 17,000   ·

      C) 25,000

9. Pesticides can remain active for _____.

      A) days

      B) weeks

      C) years

      D) all of the above

10) Of the 35,000 pesticides used in the United States, only _____ have been tested.

      A) 10 percent

      B) 25 percent

      C) 60 percent

Answers to Pesticides Quiz

1. A According to the Code of Federal Regulations 162.10, it is illegal to claim that a pesticide is safe, even if the label contains a qualifying phrase such as "when used as directed."

2. C Children have been identified as being at greater risk from pesticide exposures because they inhale more pesticides per body weight than do adults, their playing habits often put them in direct contact with residues, and their cells divide rapidly (increasing the probability of cell mutation).

3. B In spite of the fact that DDT has been banned since 1972, it can still be found on food crops. For example, Dicofol, a registered pesticide, contains up to 15 percent DDT as a contaminant. The EPA allows Dicofol to remain registered because DDT is not the "active" ingredient listed on the label.

4. B Crop losses due to insects have doubled for several reasons. First, insects develop genetic resistance to pesticides. A report from the National Academy of Sciences states that almost every major insect found in the fields is resistant to more than one type of pesticide. Second, the current use of pesticides eliminates many of the natural predators of insects. In addition, monocultural farming practices lead to crop losses. Despite the fact that one billion pounds of pesticides are used annually in the United States, an estimated 33 percent of all crops are still lost to pests each year. In contrast, alternative nonchemical methods for controlling pests have proven highly effective. For example, out of 29 million acres of alfalfa grown in the U.S., approximately 9 million acres are infested with the spotted alfalfa aphid. However, this pest has primarily been controlled by using "natural predators" and by growing alfalfa strains resistant to the aphid.

5. A   If no "alternatives" to a pesticide are known, the EPA can authorize emergency waivers for any pesticide—including those that have been previously banned. For example, in 1982 and 1983, ferriamicide, banned in 1977 because it persists in the soil and is a potential carcinogen, was granted an emergency wavier by the EPA so it could be used against fire ants in three states.

6. B   Currently, there is no legislation that prohibits U.S. companies from manufacturing unregistered, banned, or severely restricted pesticides—as long as the pesticides are intended for export. In addition, these companies do not have to provide any health and safety data on what they are producing—despite the fact that the workers in these plants, the people who load and unload the chemicals, and the rest of us who are subjected to periodic toxic spills are still being exposed to these chemicals.

7. C   Consumers have no way of monitoring whether or not pest control service applications have been properly administered unless they hire a private company to conduct post-testing. This is rarely done since these tests are very expensive.

8. B   Each year, 17,000 young children are poisoned by home pesticides. Approximately seventy million pounds of pesticides are used around the home, and more than 90 percent of these have not been properly tested for acute toxicity.

9. D   A common misconception about pesticide applications is that the pesticide is no longer harmful after it has "dried." The fact is that some pesticides have a half-life of fifty to seventy-five years (DDT, for example). In addition, pesticide residues from a variety of different applications can combine to produce an even more toxic compound.

10. A   While only 10 percent of the pesticides used in this country have ever been tested, 40 percent of the pesticides used on crops are only applied to make food "look good."

CHAPTER TWO

Pesticides in Our Lives

About a month after we moved from our toxic home to our new residence, my next door neighbor called. She wanted to inform me that her pest control service was coming the following day. Considerate of my sensitivity to pesticides, she wanted to give me advance notice so that I could make whatever arrangements I felt were necessary.

After hanging up, I debated for over an hour whether or not to call her back. At that time, I still felt that each person was entitled to live his or her own life—even if it meant spraying what I now consider to be lethal chemicals. On the other hand, I wanted her to know that there are non-chemical ways to treat pest problems. I could even refer her to a local company that specialized in completely nontoxic applications. After thinking it over, I finally decided it wouldn't hurt to make the suggestion. So I called. My neighbor listened politely to me, but said that she needed to take care of the problem immediately and believed that her pest control company could keep the ants on her patio from entering her home. She promised to consider using the nontoxic company in the future. I graciously told her that I understood and would just plan on leaving when her pest control company arrived.

I came back home the following evening and felt fine. But when I ventured into our backyard the next morning, everything changed. I had been standing near our shared fence for approximately two minutes when, suddenly, the earth below me began to spin. I would have fallen over if the person standing next to me had not caught me. For the next twenty-four hours, I continued to experience a severe reaction that included a racing heart, dizziness, weakness, eye swelling, tightening in the chest and wild mood swings. Once again, after spending six months detoxing chemicals and moving to a chemical-free home, I was completely incapacitated.

During my reaction, the same neighbor's little girl came over to play with my daughter. When she saw how sick I was, she looked quite concerned. Laying on the bed, I overheard her ask my daughter, "Why is your mommy sick?" With no malice, but in a definite matter-of-fact voice, my three-year-old responded, "My mommy's sick because your mommy sprayed."

The day before I would have cringed to hear my daughter say that. We had been extremely careful in teaching our children to keep a low profile in regards to our new beliefs towards chemicals. But that day, as I lay there with a multitude of horrendous symptoms, I no longer cared. My daughter was simply telling it like it was.

My attitude changed with that reaction. I am no longer afraid to voice my strong convictions about pesticides. The overwhelming, documented information available combined with my own personal experience leads me to one very precise statement: It is impossible to conclude that pesticide usage is safe for anyone.

Throughout this chapter, I examine safety claims made about pesticides, an important issue considering the fact that the majority of pesticides used today have either been incompletely or inaccurately tested or else have not been tested at all. The chapter also focuses on the health hazards associated with pesticides, especially for children, and the use of pesticides in food, around the home, in workplaces, and in schools. The nontoxic solutions which appear in the second half of the chapter will hopefully show the reader that there are safe and effective alternatives to chemical pest control.

THE PROBLEMS

HEALTH HAZARDS OF PESTICIDES

McFarland, California, a small town surrounded by cotton fields and almond orchards, is unremarkable except for one startling statistic: McFarland has a cancer rate four times the national average. Since 1983, six children, ranging in age from two to fifteen, have died from the deadly disease. Residents first became alarmed when two children living on the same street were diagnosed. They became even more frightened when a third child, who lived just a block away from the other two, was also diagnosed as having cancer.

Following an investigation, a preliminary report was released in February 1988 which concluded that the most probable explanation for the outbreak of cancer in this area was the *use of pesticides*.

Sadly, McFarland is only one of many areas across the country that have been identified as cancer "clusters." In addition, although cancer is one of the deadliest health problems linked to pesticide use, it is only one of many.

There is no question that pesticides are poisonous. They are specifically intended to destroy insects. One type of commonly used pesticides, organophosphates, destroys insects by disrupting their nerve impulses. The insect's nervous system becomes overloaded, and, ultimately, the insect loses nervous coordination and dies. A concern shared by many is that organophosphates do not have the ability to distinguish between insects and mammals.

Organophosphates, which are found in many pesticide formulas, are actually derived from the same family of chemicals that are used to make *nerve gas*. In fact, they originated out of chemical warfare research.

In humans, the brain and the nervous system are the two primary targets of pesticides. Depending on the individual and the type of exposure, typical symptoms include: poor memory, inability to concentrate, paresthesia (nerve tingling and numbness), anxiety, depression, hyperacusis (noises seem louder than they are), fatigue, and ataxia (poor balance).

This last symptom became apparent to me during my first visit with the clinical ecologist. I remember him asking me to stand on one foot and close my eyes. About half a second later, he had to catch me from falling over. I tried again (after all, at age thirty-three, I knew I could balance on one foot, right?), but once again, I fell over almost as soon as I closed my eyes. While I was determined to prove my ability to balance, I was really proving the doctor's belief that I had been poisoned by pesticides. The doctor explained that a person should normally be able to balance on one foot with their eyes closed for at least ten seconds. I continued to give myself this test as I detoxed, and I now can balance easily for at least thirty seconds.

Symptoms resulting from pesticide exposure may appear immediately following the exposure or *long after*. There is a difference between acute and chronic conditions. In the acute situation, the individual is exposed to a concentrated amount of pesticides for a very short period of time. The National Poison Control Center reports that it receives an estimated 100,000 calls concerning pesticide poisoning each year.

However, according to Dr. Russell Jaffe of Serammune Physicians Lab in Reston, Virginia, as many as sixteen million people may actually suffer from some form of adverse reaction to pesticides. According to his study, approximately five million people suffer from reactions severe enough to potentially result in death. Another 500,000 people are affected with asthma, bronchitis, eczema, or migraine headaches, and the remaining approximate eleven million break out in hives or suffer from muscle and joint pain.

When exposure to pesticides has been in small doses over a long period of time, the cause and effect relationship between the symptoms and the pesticide may not be obvious for a variety of reasons. First of all, pesticides are stored in body tissues. Small amounts of the stored pesticides can then slowly be released into the bloodstream over a period of months. Therefore, although a one-time exposure might be too small to be measured by a medical test, it may be enough to cause persisting symptoms.

Secondly, pesticides are known to "hit and run." In other words, they can damage crucial detoxification enzymes (discussed later) before "leaving" the body. In such cases, the pesticides themselves have been excreted, but not before adversely affecting the body's overall detoxification system. As a result, a person may then be unable to detox other common, everyday chemicals. This "hit and run" nature of pesticides is of particular concern since many traditional doctors do not believe that low-level exposures to pesticides can cause chronic health conditions or damage the detoxification system. As a result, many pesticide-related health conditions may go undiagnosed or misdiagnosed. I must have asked at least seven of the twenty traditional doctors I saw in the early months of my decline if the pesticides sprayed in my home could be affecting my breathing. I was told over and over again, "Absolutely not."

HEALTH HAZARDS FOR CHILDREN

As dangerous as pesticides can be to adults, they can pose an even *greater* threat to children. Many experts claim that children are at a much higher risk of pesticide poisoning than adults. One basic reason for this is that in relation to body weight, children inhale or ingest a greater percentage of toxins than adults do. In addition, test studies show that children have lower levels of the enzymes needed by the body to rid itself of toxins naturally.

Children under the age of five also have a faster respiratory rate than adults, which means they inhale more chemicals than adults. And since children tend to breathe more through their mouths, many of the residues which might otherwise be trapped in the nasal passages make their way to the lungs. Once in the lungs toxic substances can injure lung tissue and be absorbed into the bloodstream.

The playing habits of children also place them in more direct contact with pesticide residues. Children typically somersault on carpets, run barefoot on lawns, or dig through dirt—activities which increase the likelihood of a child being exposed to pesticides. In addition, most parents who employ a pest control service are not concerned when their children later play on areas that have been sprayed after the waiting period suggested by the pest control service is over. I know I thought nothing of letting my babies crawl on our carpet shortly after our home had been sprayed. I never thought to question how the pest control companies determined how long the waiting period should be. Nor did I question how the pesticide residues could be strong enough to kill pests in my home for months but not strong enough to affect me or my family just a few hours later or during the following months.

There are other physiological differences between children and adults that also account for a pesticide's greater affect on children. The cell activity and organ development of children differs from adults. In early childhood, cells divide more rapidly. This rapid division increases the likelihood of cell mutations and the subsequent risk of cancer. Studies have also shown that children's immature digestive systems allow them to absorb more toxic chemicals. The immaturity of other organs can further make children more susceptible to health hazards.

For example, since a child's brain continues to develop after birth, it is even more likely to be affected by neurotoxins. The brain is most susceptible to toxins during the developmental stage called myelination. During myelination, nerve fibers are covered with a fat-like substance. The most rapid phase of myelination is completed by age two—yet, myelination does not totally end until adolescence. Young children are also more sensitive to neurotoxins because their nerve fibers are still branching.

A final concern is the possible relationship between pesticides and the serious children's illness called Reye's Syndrome. This illness, which can lead to rapid liver failure, coma, and death, is believed to follow certain viral infections, specifically the flu. A study done by Dr. Crocker at Dalhouse University has linked Reye's Syndrome to pesticide poisoning. Prompted by an outbreak of the disease following an aerial pesticide spraying, Dr. Crocker constructed an experimental model with laboratory mice to study the effect of pesticides. In the experiment, some mice were exposed to the insecticides, some were exposed to the influenza virus, and some to both. A number of the mice treated with the insecticides died, as did a number of the mice inoculated with the virus. However, *all* of the mice that were exposed to both the insecticides and the virus died of an illness similar to Reye's Syndrome.[3]

PESTICIDES IN FOOD

If you think as I used to, you have probably given little thought to what chemicals may have been applied to the produce we eat. However, the next time you decide to have a nice, healthy salad for lunch, keep in mind that *thirty* different pesticides have been detected in carrots alone.

Despite the fact that DDT has been banned since 1972 because of its toxicity, DDT residues were found in 17 percent of domestic carrots in a recent survey. DDT can still be detected in food crops because it still persists in the environment and the soil.

Equally disturbing is the repeated detection of dieldrin in carrots. Dieldrin is known to cause birth defects and reproductive toxicity in animal studies. Even low levels have caused learning disabilities in monkeys. As with DDT, the use of dieldrin has been banned by the EPA since 1974, but residues persist in food crops.

Carrots are not to be singled out. *Every non-organic fruit and vegetable may contain multiple numbers of pesticide residues.*

Actress Meryl Streep and the Natural Resource Defense Council brought concern about pesticide residues in food to the national forefront when they claimed that Alar, a common chemical applied to apples, was toxic.

In response to the alarm about Alar and the growing concern about pesticide residues in food in general, many parents now take extra care in washing their produce. However, in most cases, washing produce will *not* eliminate pesticide residues for several reasons. First, most pesticides are specifically formulated to be water resistant since farmers and growers do not want their pesticide application to be washed away with the first rain. Second, many pesticides are systemic, making any outside scrubbing futile.

In addition, produce that has been waxed also poses a concern since waxing seals in pesticide residues, to say nothing of the fungicide which has been added to the wax itself.

While most consumers may know that cucumbers are waxed, they may not know that a number of other fruits and vegetables are also routinely waxed. These include apples, avocados, bell peppers, cantaloupes, eggplants, grapefruits, lemons, limes, melons, oranges, parsnips, passion fruits, peaches, pineapples, pumpkins, rutabagas, squash, sweet potatoes, and turnips.

Pesticide residues are more likely to be found in produce which has a high standard for cosmetic appearance or if the edible portion of the produce is in direct contact with the soil when it is grown. Such produce includes strawberries, peaches, celery, cherries, cucumbers, bell peppers, and tomatoes.

Imported Food

Not all produce has the same amount of pesticide residues. In one study, which examined inspections of produce done between 1983 and 1985, *im-*

ported food showed higher traces of pesticides (almost double) than foods grown domestically.[4] Even more disturbing is the *type* of pesticides that were found.

When I first began researching pesticide application and usage, I was alarmed to discover that the more commonly used pesticides in Third World countries are either *unregistered*, *banned*, or *severely restricted* in the United States. Despite the proven hazards of these pesticides, current law allows U.S. companies to manufacture them as long as they are exported.

But this illogical injustice does not just affect families in the Third World. Up to 70 percent of the food grown abroad with the aid of unregistered, banned or severely restricted pesticides is exported back into this country.[5] Much of the food on the shelves of your local grocery store was grown with the help of these hazardous pesticides. The fact that so much of the food grown abroad gets exported back to this country calls into question the argument that hazardous pesticides are desperately needed by Third World countries so that they can grow food to alleviate hunger.

American families are further subjected to the hazards of these chemicals as long as U.S. companies that manufacture pesticides for export are not legally required to provide health and safety data on what they are actually producing. Workers in these plants—people who load and unload the chemicals onto trucks, ships, planes, or trains—and those who are exposed to toxic spills all become part of the shared, worldwide problem of the legal export of untested or confirmed hazardous pesticides.

PEST CONTROL AROUND THE HOME

Approximately 91 percent of all Americans use some type of pest control and/or lawn care chemicals around the home. In fact, approximately 1.5 billion dollars are spent yearly on lawn care alone. Yet, what are these chemicals and how safe are they?

As an example, let's consider diazinon, a common organophosphate insecticide used in and around the home. This pesticide inhibits the enzyme cholinesterase (ChE). This can lead to respiratory arrest, paralysis, convulsions, and even death. Milder forms of diazinon poisoning can cause chest tightening, decreased heart beat, nausea, twitching, headache, and dizziness.

In April 1986, a review of diazinon testing data by the California Department of Food and Agriculture revealed that there were no adequate tests on file. In other words, despite the fact that this pesticide can be bought and used by any consumer, no test for cancer, chronic effects, birth defects, reproductive effects, or gene damage were on record.

Like other pesticides, diazinon can become highly concentrated in fog.

For example, it was found present in fog in California in concentrations 1,100 times greater than expected. It has also been found in open bodies of water and groundwater in forty-six states.

Diazinon is certainly not the only pesticide used by consumers. In fact, one is almost guaranteed to find common, commercial bug sprays in most homes. However, because these products can be bought at the grocery store, I fear that most people do not really comprehend that these too are PESTI-CIDES with significant health hazards. For example, the active ingredient in one commercial roach control product is chlorpyrifos, which is known to produce neurotoxic effects in humans, including learning disabilities. My personal alarm goes off when I hear this because I now know that chlor-pyrifos is the same active ingredient used in the pesticide formulation ap-plied to my home.

Pest Control Companies

Then there are those (like myself before my illness) who don't want to be personally bothered with getting rid of pests. These people hire a pest con-trol service to do the work instead.

We certainly thought that a service was a great solution to our flea and ant problem. Unfortunately, I had no idea that if a house has been sprayed even once within the last twenty years pesticide residues may continue to linger. It is known that Dursban, the product used in my home, can linger for ten to fifteen years, while chlordane residues, which can even pass through plastic packaging in freezers and have been detected in freezer doors and the rubber parts of refrigerators, will remain for as long as twenty-five to thirty-five years.

If we had been thinking about pesticide safety at all back then, we should have at least become suspicious of the obvious discrepancies between the various companies we employed. For example, even though all three of the pest control companies we used emphatically (and I now know illegally) claimed that their applications were safe, each gave us different advice on how to handle our dog while the spraying took place. Company A told us it was fine for our dog to remain in the yard during the application; Company B put the dog in the garage during the exterior spraying but immediately re-turned it to the yard during the interior application; and Company C in-formed us that the dog must be off the premises the entire time the house was sprayed and closed.

The amount of time the family had to wait before returning to the house also varied among companies, ranging anywhere between two to four hours. In addition, the pest service employees seemed to set higher safety standards for themselves than they did for their customers. On one occasion, a service person began spraying our yard before my children and I had a chance to leave the vicinity. He was wearing a mask; we, of course, were not.

Likewise, most people who employ a pesticide service are not on a first name basis with their exterminators. I know I certainly never knew any of the various individuals that came to my home. Yet, I entrusted these perfect strangers to enter my residence and spray toxic materials. I guess I just assumed that these strangers were conscious, responsible workers who were incapable of making any "on-the-job" errors.

This assumption now seems completely ridiculous to me. All workers—not to single out exterminators—have both good and bad days at work and their share of job-related errors. Therefore, even those who strongly believe that pesticide applications are safe in designated amounts cannot ignore the variable of the "serviceperson." These individuals can only hope that their home is serviced with the correct application.

In addition, most pest control companies have a policy that actually encourages overspraying. This policy allows consumers to request that the company return to spray once again—free of charge—if the pest problem does not improve within the time period agreed upon between the company and customer. This "gratis" return visit, however, can transform your most casual serviceperson into a zealous baseboard bomber—to please you and to make sure the company does not have to return again.

After our own "gratis" application, the pesticide smell lingered for nearly *three* weeks, despite round the clock airing of the house. It was during this time that I went from being merely ill to being completely incapacitated and unable to breathe.

One year later, I casually mentioned to another pest control employee, who was inspecting our home to satisfy escrow requirements for its sale, how I thought that return visit may have been an "overkill" application. While I had actually come to believe this, I still wasn't prepared for his response. Vigorously nodding his head, the serviceperson not only agreed, but even made a point of telling me, "Oh yeah, they really nuke you on those return visits."

"Overkill" does not happen just in homes; many places of business also rely on routine pesticide applications. Since I began researching this book, I am not sure if more incidents of pesticide oversprayings are happening or if I am just more aware of this possibility. For example, over 100 people were recently evacuated from Pacific Bell's Irvine, California, office. Of these 100, 40 were treated for chemical exposure at local hospitals with symptoms that included severe headache, shortness of breath, faintness, nausea, burning eyes, sore throats, and heart arrhythmias. Over the weekend the office had been sprayed by a local company for "paper fleas."

After two days of intensive office cleaning after the incident, Bell employees still claimed that they noticed a lingering diazinon odor. I know from my own personal experience that continual inhalation of pesticides after the body has already become sensitized or weakened (e.g., from an overspraying) can slowly turn into a serious, chronic health condition.

Oversprayings can occur outside homes too. A neighbor of mine who sprayed shortly after we had moved in became concerned for her own family's health when my husband pointed out to her that the exterior of her home still smelled of the chemical forty-eight hours after its application. Confused, she called the company and asked how long the smell should linger by their standards. The company's response was two to three hours for outdoor applications. Therefore, by the company's own admission, something had to be wrong. But what? An incorrect mixture of chemicals? A spill? An overspraying? Any or all of these may have been the cause.

Entomophobia

I have spent a long time trying to figure out why some people, in spite of all the available information, still insist on using pesticides. Sometimes I feel like Columbus when he KNEW the world was round, but the majority was still convinced it was flat. I *really* have tried to convince my neighbors who spray that their repeated applications of pesticides are harmful, but I have yet to find many believers. I still see numerous pesticide trucks stop regularly in front of various homes on my block. But, when I see the trucks, I don't think that my neighbors are "bad people." On the contrary, I do not think I could live by kinder or friendlier people. I truthfully do not think that any of my neighbors or friends believe I have fabricated my symptoms and story, and I am certainly convinced that they are genuinely concerned and dedicated when it comes to the well-being of their children. So I think something more powerful than facts and first-hand knowledge of someone's personal experience continues to draw them to pesticides—over and over again.

I believe I may have found an explanation: entomophobia, the unreasonable fear of insects and like creatures. It actually is a condition, and it might explain why my neighbors have even refused our offer to pay for a nontoxic pest control service for them. Perhaps these people become so distressed when they see a few ants or other pests about to approach their home that they believe the only solution is to immediately exterminate them, with the most lethal approach available.

For example, recently some of our surrounding neighbors insisted that they once again had a pest problem and, therefore, *had* to call in their pest control company. My husband and I found it incredibly interesting that our spraying neighbors had another ant problem, when we (who have never sprayed in our current home) had no problem at all. Based on that information alone, it could be that repeated pesticide applications actually encourage long-term pest problems. This thought reinforced what we had come to realize long ago: it was probably never in a pest control company's best interest to truly control pests—if they did they would soon be out of business.

We also wondered whether or not our neighbors really did have a pest *problem* or if just a few ants had entered their homes. However, they explained to us that there were ants in the cereal and that some flowers were dying (even though it was November). There was no doubt in their minds that the service was needed.

For the present, all I am able to do when they decide to spray is to close my windows and sigh deeply. But I always find myself tempted to ask them, "What do you think is the worst thing that could happen if you could not use pesticides? Is it that *several* boxes of cereal might become infested with ants? Is it that a portion of your grass will turn brown? Is it that your yard will have a few less flowers?"

I cannot even imagine their answers. *My* worst nightmare would be to hear that my child had leukemia (children exposed to household poisons have a *seven* times greater chance of getting leukemia, according to one study) after I had been warned about the established connection between pesticides and cancer.

PESTICIDES IN SCHOOLS

Health-related Incidents

As a fifth grade teacher, I can clearly remember one rainy morning in my classroom. My thirty students were earnestly simplifying fractions while the school's custodian was busily spraying the baseboard for ants. Looking back, I recall no policy that dictated when, if, or how the custodian was authorized to eliminate the ants. As a teacher, while I was required to fill out countless forms for just about everything, I remember no procedure for having one's room sprayed. In fact, I believe I merely "buzzed" the front office and requested that my ants be zapped.

Considering the amount of time children spend in schools, coupled with children's increased risk of pesticide-related illness, the use of pesticides in schools is a very important, often overlooked, issue. Since I began my research, I have become aware of many incidents where routine pesticide applications at schools turned into nightmares for unsuspecting students. For example, in Yakima, Washington, a seven-year-old boy ate a pinch of "sand" beneath a maple tree on his school playground. However, the "sand" was actually a highly toxic pesticide, and the child nearly lost his life.

In another elementary school in Hawaii, twenty-eight students and three faculty members developed headaches, stomach aches, breathing difficulties, and nausea after their school was treated for a flea problem with the commonly-used pesticide Dursban. As a result, all students and staff were sent home, and the school had to remain closed the following day.

However, not surprisingly, the fleas remained a problem at this elementary school despite massive pesticide treatments. It is unfortunate that the school has not implemented a preventive strategy (e.g., fencing) to prevent dogs, the probable source of the fleas, from sleeping underneath the portable classrooms. Not only would this be more effective, but it would undeniably be a much safer solution for the children and the staff.

If these were only two isolated incidents, there would still be plenty of justification for concern; unfortunately, the list goes on. Twenty students and six staff members at a high school in Oregon complained of various symptoms after exterminators applied Dursban to control termites in their school. Twenty-four Chicago high school students suffered severe nausea, dizziness, headaches and other symptoms the day after they were exposed to a roach killer. In Charleston, West Virginia, a junior high school was finally closed after four years of complaints by students and teachers of persistent fatigue, headaches, nausea, respiratory problems, and numbness in the limbs. Investigators for the National Institute of Occupational Safety and Health (NIOSH) found the school to be contaminated with chlordane. In fact, the investigators found the chlordane levels in the school's air to be eleven times higher than the limit at which the National Academy of Sciences (NAS) recommends a school to evacuate its premises.

Policy

Unfortunately, pesticide policy is still not likely to be a leading issue in most schools. Currently, the two major teacher unions have not expressed a formal position on this issue, allowing pest control policies to vary from district to district. A survey conducted by the Better Government Association revealed that twenty-one of thirty-eight Chicago area school districts responded that they apply pesticides at least once a month. Similar responses were given in surveys across the nation. Moreover, this routine spraying is also more than likely being done without parent notification (let alone consent). This fact continually amazes me since as a teacher I was not even allowed to give a child a single aspirin without parental permission. Yet, it seems highly improbable that a school district would call a parent and say the following: *"Hello, Mrs. Garcia. I'm calling to inform you that we will be subjecting your child to a product whose primary ingredient has not yet been tested for adverse health affects (or was, in fact, fraudulently tested). As for the other ingredients (the inert ingredients), I'm sorry, but we cannot tell you anything about them because we actually haven't the faintest idea what they are. I guess we're just hoping that this product doesn't contain any of the fifty-five commonly used inerts that are known to be of toxicological concern. But be reassured though, we do know something—the primary purpose of this product is to kill."*

Applications

Parents might be under the false assumption that pesticides are only applied to schools when the students are not present. This is not true. Yet, even applying pesticides on the weekends, when students are not there, does not resolve the problem of possible hazardous consequences resulting from the applications. Many pesticides are intentionally designed to have long residual effects to kill pests over a period of several weeks or months. School classrooms contain many porous materials, such as rugs, books, and plastics, to which pesticide residues can bind, further delaying the breakdown process. In addition, the creation of year-round schools in many districts has subsequently eliminated summer as the "safe" months for heavy chemical applications.

Another problem is that pesticides may be applied by non-certified personnel. By law, each state determines requirements for certification for access to certain chemicals. Typically, applicants attend a multi-week class and must pass a written exam. However, a loophole in the law allows non-certified applicators to use the pesticides under the supervision of a certified person. The direct result of this loophole is that many custodians who are responsible for the sprayings at the school sites have received no certified training.

One of the causes of overuse of pesticides in schools is that they are usually applied according to some pre-established schedule—regardless of whether or not the pests are even present at the time of application. In addition, crisis management, as opposed to implementing preventative measures, lends itself to overuse and dependency on toxic chemicals.

Moreover, the *type* of pesticides commonly used at schools is also of great concern. For example, 2,4D is used on some school lawns and athletic fields despite the fact that it is a component of the banned, notorious Agent Orange. In a Federal District Court, a jury awarded the family of a deceased forestry worker 1.5 million dollars after concluding that 2,4D was linked to the worker's death. ChemLawn, one of the country's largest lawn care companies, stopped using 2,4D after a recent study by the National Cancer Institute linked 2,4D with certain cancers among Kansas farmers. However, neither of these actions has prevented 2,4D from being applied on school grounds.

Treatment of Lice

Parents are sometimes actually *encouraged* to put their children in direct contact with pesticides. A study done by the National Pediculosis Association (NPA) reported that an alarming number of schools are sending parents notifications on how to treat their children's head lice. The suggested treatments include indiscriminate environmental spraying (instead of careful vacuuming) and recommendations for the use of a lindane-based pediculicide (instead of a less toxic product) on the entire family, not just the infested child.

Anyone who works in a school or who has children is very aware that head lice can be a real problem. In fact, one can expect anywhere from 3 to 5 percent of the children within a school to be infested with head lice at any given time. Therefore, it is not surprising that over forty million dollars were spent in 1987 on pesticides for human lice treatment.

However, the typically recommended lindane-based shampoos are very toxic and dangerous to children. Like other chlorinated hydrocarbons (such as DDT), *lindane* penetrates the skin, enters the bloodstream, and then is eventually stored in the body's organs and/or tissues. Once there, it can accumulate and is capable of producing neurotoxicity when it reaches sufficient concentrations in the blood or brain tissue. Considering that applications for treating lice require direct contact with the scalp, these established facts trigger great concern.

It should also be noted that even using a pediculicide without a lindane-base is hazardous since *all lice treatments on the market today are made from some kind of pesticide.*

COMPLICATING FACTORS

Many factors are involved in determining pesticide safety. For example, there exists only incomplete or inaccurate testing data on many pesticides and virtually no data is available to the public on the health hazards of inert ingredients. Another concern is the fact that economic considerations are very influential in determining whether or not a pesticide will be allowed on the market. Two other factors which cloud the pesticide safety issue are illegal safety claims by pesticide companies and false advertising.

Incomplete and/or Inaccurate Testing

It is difficult to conclude that pesticides are safe when one reviews how these chemicals are tested, what has actually been tested (and what has not), and who is doing the testing.

The EPA and FDA rely heavily on *industry-sponsored* research and testing to determine the potential health risks of pesticides. Concern over unbiased and inaccurate testing was highlighted in 1981 when the owners of Industrial Bio-test Labs were prosecuted and sent to prison after the EPA found that over 90 percent of more than 2,000 studies on pesticides submitted by the lab were falsified and invalid.[6] However, as of mid-1984, less than 243 of the pesticides had been reevaluated. In fact, the EPA has now decided to wait until the rest of the chemicals in question go through the EPA's normal process of review, which, due to a severe staff shortage and continual cutbacks, is not likely to happen for a very long time. In short, despite the fact that fraudulent testing has been undeniably confirmed, the majority of the products whose registrations were dependent upon Industrial Bio-test Lab results are still on the market and are being used daily.

Additionally, the primary emphasis of industry-sponsored research is on determining which pesticides cause cancer. Although this is important research, little time or money is spent on studying the relationship between pesticides and damage to the immune system and neurological and psychological disorders; the increased susceptibility of children, the elderly, or adults with chronic health problems; or the synergistic effects of exposures to multiple pesticide residues. These are important issues that also need to be addressed.

Presently, only one very limited test is even required by the EPA to determine the potential neurotoxic effects of pesticides in humans. This test focuses solely on what levels of exposures may cause paralysis and death. The EPA requires no testing on how acute and chronic exposures affect motor coordination, learning disabilities, or memory. However, various independent studies have concluded that exposure to organophosphates may greatly alter and affect nerve transmission and neuromuscular function, neuroreceptor development, and brain electrical activity.

The Problem with Safety Claims

Claims that pesticides are safe are often based on the scientific lethal dose (LD_{50}) of a pesticide. Anything below this lethal dose is considered "safe." However, the LD_{50} figure merely shows the dose at which 50 percent of the animals tested die. By this criterion, a dose that kills as many as 49 percent is still considered safe.

The No Observable Effect Level (NOEL) is used to "prove" that a pesticide is harmless below a certain dosage. However, the NOEL simply means that in one particular test researchers did not find the effect *that they were looking for* in the species they were testing. Using the NOEL as the measure of pesticide safety does not take into account the fact that other methods of observation, different kinds of exposures, or observation of a different organ (e.g., liver damage versus kidney) may, indeed, produce very different results.

Flaws in Food Safety Claims

As unbelievable as it might seem, all of our current pesticides introduced before 1977 have undergone no testing for carcinogenicity, mutagenicity, teratogenicity, or infertility effects. These pesticides are exempt from testing since they came onto the market prior to EPA regulations mandating industry testing of chemicals for health hazards.

Another flaw in food safety claims becomes evident when examining the EPA's level of legal pesticide residues. To begin with, the EPA used a 125-pound person as its model of the average consumer. Not only does the EPA testing not compensate for persons of lesser or greater weights, but it also does not account for the specific dietary habits of children.

Moreover, these "tolerable" levels, the levels at which ingestion of a pesticide is believed to pose minimal or no health risks to humans, were established in the late 1960s. However, these levels do not take into consideration our increased consumption of produce over the past decades. For example, the EPA assumes that we eat no more than half a pound *per year* of artichokes, avocados, blueberries, blackberries, cantaloupe, honeydew melon, eggplant, plums, tangerines, nectarines, or radishes. By the EPA's own standards, consumers who eat more than half a pound of these foods are potentially exposed to more pesticide residues than the agency considers safe. Additionally, tolerance levels were also established with the erroneous assumption that a person would only be exposed to the pesticide once in a lifetime. The EPA does not calculate the total number of times a person has been exposed. Nor does it consider the multiple pesticides applied to food crops. The whole premise of "tolerance levels" is simply based on theoretical assumptions.

Additionally, no one can accurately determine the extent of food contamination by pesticide residues since over one-half of the pesticides being applied to food crops cannot even be detected by routine laboratory methods. Also, only about 1 percent of our food is actually sampled.[7] However, detection of high or illegal pesticide residues still does not necessarily prevent the contaminated food from reaching the consumer. For example, in 1986, a Los Angeles laboratory detected illegal pesticide residues in at least six shipments of Mexican cantaloupes. However, two of these shipments were still sold in the United States because the FDA allows some shipments of perishable foods to be sold prior to obtaining the results of the sample analysis.

After I became aware of these flaws in food safety claims, I wrote a letter to the FDA to express my concerns over pesticide residues. To my surprise, I actually received a response, but the response was quite predictable.

Two long handouts accompanied the brief note acknowledging my letter. It was obvious that these handouts had been prepared to respond to the countless letters that I imagine the agency must now receive. The handouts explain in great detail, with numerous statistics, just how safe our food is. Their facts are impressive, and a person without any additional knowledge in this area might conclude that his or her concerns about food safety are unwarranted. After all, the handout points out that the FDA has been monitoring foods for pesticides for over twenty-five years. The agency assures the reader that the residues found in foods are generally far below EPA tolerance levels.

But what concerns me are the facts the FDA chose *not* to include. The FDA knows that it only tests about 1 percent of the food sold. It knows, too, that more than half of the pesticides used on food crops cannot be detected by routine laboratory methods. The agency also knows that the EPA tolerance levels referred to extensively in the handout were established several decades ago and do not take into account the dietary habits of children. Last of all, the agency is aware that current testing of pesticides and food has not focused on chronic health problems or the synergistic effects when multiple pesticides are used. Yet, the FDA did not include any of this information in its handout.

To me, by presenting only selected facts and statistics, the agency risks losing credibility. A fair report would have included both the agency's findings *and* the limitations currently associated with monitoring pesticides.

Inert Ingredients and Loopholes

Pesticides contain two types of ingredients—active and inert. Active ingredients, which are listed on a product's label, are those which are intended to kill the targeted organism. Inert ingredients are virtually everything else in the product; they are not listed on the label since they are considered to be "trade secrets." Sometimes less than a teaspoon of the active ingredient can be fatal to a 200-pound man; therefore, a liquid vehicle composed from an inert ingredient is needed. Commonly used inert ingredients are acetone, asbestos, benzene, toluene, phenol, xylene, dioxin, formaldehyde, and tetrachloride—all of which are considered toxic.

Presently, the law requires that tests be conducted to determine the potential health hazards of active ingredients only. It is not required that the inert ingredients be tested, even though they often comprise as much as 90 to 99 percent of the total product. Approximately 1,200 trade secret inert ingredients have never been tested, nor are they scheduled to be reviewed at any time. Of this 1,200, there is virtually no available information on 800 of these ingredients; 55 have been established to be of serious toxicological concern.[8]

The inert ingredients of a formula can greatly affect those who are exposed to the pesticide containing the inert. In May 1987, a faculty member of Oregon State University became ill following a brief exposure to Diazinon PT-260, which had been sprayed into a crack in the office in which she worked. It is difficult to pinpoint the chemical that triggered her severe response because Diazinon PT-260 is composed of only 1 percent diazinon and 99 *percent inert ingredients*. After an investigation, it was disclosed that methylene chloride and 1, 1, 1-trichloromethane compose the bulk of this "diazinon" formula. Methylene chloride, a neurotoxin, is a mutagen (causing gene damage) and a possible carcinogen (causing cancer); 1, 1, 1-trichloromethane is a possible carcinogen.

Another concern with inert ingredients in pesticide formulas is with aerial applications of pesticides such as malathion. In communities that employ aerial spraying of pesticides, workers and community residents are informed of the pesticide application. However, the workers and residents have no way of knowing that the pesticide formulations may also contain benzene, formaldehyde, or any number of toxic inert ingredients.

Many pesticide manufacturers may themselves not even be able to identify the inert ingredients they use in their products since they can buy formulas "blindly" from an inert chemical manufacturer. This makes it impossible for the EPA to even request manufacturers to flag which of their pesticides contain any of the fifty-five hazardous inerts since the manufacturers may not know themselves.

While the EPA does have a list of the majority of inert ingredients used in pesticide formulations, the list is given very little (if any) consideration. This point was confirmed when an EPA staff member discovered that DDT (which has been banned since 1972) is used as an inert ingredient in numerous registered pesticides currently in use.[9] In some cases, even the EPA does not know what inerts are in a pesticide. This is due to either a lack of information in the "file" or because during the 1972 petroleum shortage the EPA issued a notice allowing registrants to purchase scarce solvents and emulsifiers and then list alternatives in their formula statements.[10]

Mary O'Brien, a scientist who received the 1989 Robert Bosch Memorial award for "scientific expertise and important contribution to pesticide policy improvements," sums up these concerns, "Anybody who claims to know about the safety of a pesticide formulation, the ingredients which are unidentified or untested, is either being delusional or dishonest."

False Advertising

Pesticide advertising can be both misleading and false. Many consumers are reassured by the statement "EPA registered." However, this claim does not mean that the EPA has determined the pesticide to be safe. "EPA registered" simply means that the product was registered prior to the new 1977 guidelines or that it became registered thereafter because its perceived benefits outweigh the *known* risks. Pesticides are not registered because they have been *proven* to pose *no* safety hazards to the public. In fact, the EPA states "because pesticides are by their very nature designed to be biologically active and kill pests and weeds, we speak in terms of relative risks, rather than safety. The introduction of toxic chemicals into the environment does create both known and unknown risks to human health and environment."

Economic Considerations

The EPA sets standards which are based on the need for an "adequate, wholesome, and economical food supply." Therefore, the EPA must weigh health risks against economic gains when determining "safe" food. Health factors are not their sole consideration.

While it may not actually prove anything, citizens may find it interesting to note that from 1981 to 1986 the 6.5 billion dollar pesticide industry contributed more than 1.2 million dollars to members of the United States Senate and House agricultural committees. My guess is that it was not to promote organic farming.

The Problem with Expert Opinions

When assessing the risks associated with pesticides, there has rarely been discussion as to whether or not pesticides are potentially hazardous. Rather, the discussion centers around the different assessments of what amount of a pesticide can be inhaled or ingested without prompting adverse health consequences.

Many scientists claim that results found in animal studies are not applicable to humans. Other experts argue that by ignoring and invalidating animal studies, consumers then become the "test" animals.

Since scientists are the experts most often quoted in the media, it seems relevant to note that many of the ones who are quoted are employed by chemical companies, a fact that is often omitted or overlooked by the media. The fact that chemical companies have great financial interest in reassuring the public of chemical safety does not necessarily negate the validity of the scientist's opinion. But it does raise a concern as to whether predisposed biases exist or whether scientists might fear losing their job if they say that a chemical their company manufactures poses a health risk to humans.

Even within the EPA itself there appears to be punitive action taken against scientists who do not toe the line. For example, Adrian Gross, a senior scientist in the EPA's Hazardous Evaluation Division, was demoted a week after he wrote a forty-eight page memo accusing his superiors of illegally assisting two major chemical companies in registering a pesticide considered by Gross to be a "potent carcinogen." His new position deprived him of any access to the EPA's health and safety files.

Hugh Kaufman, a toxic waste expert within the EPA, was docked two days pay and tailed by the agency's Inspector General's Office after telling a congressional subcommittee that if he were a Soviet agent trying to poison America, he would not change the U.S. hazardous waste program one iota. On "60 Minutes," Kaufman also stated that the "EPA is not about to protect you if your state or local government won't." Four House subcommittees have been assigned to investigate whether or not the EPA is harassing Kaufman because of his outspokenness.[11]

Other scientists in agencies other than the EPA have also faced similar treatment. Melvin Reuber became a "former" scientist for the National Cancer Institute after he mailed an unpublished article on the carcinogenesis of malathion to a California environmental group that had been verbalizing its concern over the use of the pesticide in urban areas to control the Mediterranean fruit fly. He was strongly reprimanded for his actions.

On a personal level, I became aware of this potential scientist/employer conflict when Mary and Carl (a couple with whom I had become acquainted at the detox clinic) related the following story to me.

Forced to move out of their home after one of their pest control sprayings produced almost immediate ill-health in both of them, Mary and Carl extracted a promise from the pest control company to send technical experts out to determine if the home was truly contaminated from a misapplication.

As the men arrived and carried out their inspection, Mary waited outside. A short time later, the men joined her. Reassuring her that nothing was wrong, they even made a point of exclaiming what a lovely home it would be to live in.

Persistent in her belief of contamination, Mary then challenged them to return inside and actually put their noses to the carpet. One of the men accepted the challenge. According to Mary's account, he immediately came running out of the house sneezing with red and watery eyes. However, the inspector still insisted that the home was not contaminated. He claimed he was reacting to mere dust.

Feeling extremely frustrated and defeated, Mary did not know what to think. Then, one of the men pulled her aside before leaving. He told her that under no circumstances would he ever testify in court nor would he even admit that their conversation had taken place, but he wanted to inform her that her home was, indeed, very contaminated. The best he could do was to encourage her to seek an independent company to confirm the unquestionable contamination. He, however, was going to report that the house was fine because he simply could not afford to lose his job.

After a private company inspected the home, it was immediately condemned by the Board of Health.

SOLUTIONS AND ALTERNATIVES

For each of the problems with pesticides thus presented, alternatives do exist. However, they only become solutions if people are willing to try them.

ORGANIC FOOD

The concern over pesticide residues in food gained national attention in 1989 after a "60 Minutes" story on the findings and recommendations of the Natural Resource Defense Council regarding apples and the chemical Alar. The report caused a national scare. Suddenly, apples were poison. In response to the hysteria, the media printed several stories which reprimanded parents for eliminating "good" produce out of fear of pesticide residues. It appeared that parents were faced with only two choices—life with pesticide-contaminated produce or life without produce. However, many were ignoring "Door Number Three," a logical, healthy choice which included all the produce but none of the pesticides—simply, organic food.

Just the mere mention of the word organic seems to trigger different responses in various people: "Too expensive." "Too hard to find." "Food with worms."

However, these reactions usually come from people who have not even tried organic food. For example, a friend of ours and his seventeen-year-old son visited us shortly after we had switched to eating only organic food. Prior to the visit, our friend informed his son that they would be eating organic food at our home. Very concerned, the son wanted to know if that meant he would be living on "sprouts" the entire visit.

After they arrived, the first meal with our visiting friends consisted of soup, bread, and a variety of sauteed vegetables baked in zucchini shells. Not wanting to be rude, the father did not tell us that his son did not ordinarily eat vegetables—but to his surprise, the son devoured the entire meal and every meal we served after that! The father finally concluded that the organic food simply tasted better.

However, it is true that organic food is not always as accessible as other food. If necessary, groups of community residents can successfully influence traditional grocery stores to add organic food to their shelves and bins. Successful approaches for obtaining pesticide-free food have included meetings with produce managers, writing letters to the corporate management, and supplying store personnel with lists of organic growers. Additionally, many organic grains, legumes, and other non-perishable products can be easily purchased through the mail (see Appendix 2 for addresses).

Whether or not organic food costs more depends on an individual's perspective of what one is getting for the money. One of our family's priorities now is to eat good, pure food. With that perspective, it becomes irrelevant if the organic apple is twice the price of that sprayed and waxed thing also called an "apple." For us, shopping organically *is* the better bargain. Clearly, I could shop organically for the rest of my life and still spend less than I did on medical expenses during my illness. We would rather have to spend a little more on organic food now than have to spend a *lot* more on medical expenses in the future.

It should be noted, though, that the word "organic" is thus far only legally defined in three states. In California, it has been defined as food that is "produced, harvested, distributed, stored, processed, and packaged without the application of synthetically compounded fertilizers, pesticides, or growth regulators." This definition is very different from foods advertised solely as "pesticide free."

While it is commendable that some major grocery chains are attempting to address the public's concern over food safety by offering "pesticide-free" produce, consumers should understand the difference between this food and certified organic food. "Pesticide-free" signifies that upon a random inspection of the food at the dock where the food was received, no pesticides were detected. However, since more than half of the pesticides applied to crops cannot be detected by routine methods and since there is the possibility that the food will be contaminated further on down the line (before reaching the grocery shelves), "pesticide-free" does not guarantee that the food is truly without pesticides. In contrast, food that has been certified as organic is grown on farms that do not use pesticides.

Realistically, though, even certified organic food may still not be completely pure. The food can become contaminated unintentionally by neighboring farms that use chemicals, by a contaminated water supply, by airborne pesticides from nearby dust cropping, or by chemical fertilizers already in the ground. However, certified organic food is *significantly* less contaminated (if at all) than food that has been intentionally and routinely sprayed, gassed, waxed, and/or dyed.

Last of all, not only is organic food healthier and the result of better ecological farming, but it is DELICIOUS too! After eating only organic food for some time, my husband went out to lunch with his parents at a restaurant that he had always liked. While his parents enjoyed their meal, my husband found his food tasteless, "lifeless and dead." Or, in other words, processed, sprayed, and definitely not organic.

I know not everyone is going to eat only organic food. But even if you do not choose to switch to buying organic food, there are many things that you can do to reduce your exposure to pesticides in commercial food. First, with canned food, wash the can before opening; when you do open the can, open it from the bottom. This will help eliminate pesticide residues from repeated grocery store sprayings. Second, ask your supermarket to label the origin of its produce. Then, buy only domestically-grown produce to avoid food grown with the aid of exported, banned pesticides. However, note that domestic food does not include food grown in Hawaii, which is fumigated when shipped to the mainland. Lastly, buy only produce that is in season, and beware of the "perfect" or "flawless" fruit or vegetable. Chances are pesticides were applied to achieve perfection and/or to make out-of-season produce available at all times of the year.

NONTOXIC PEST CONTROL

There are a variety of nontoxic alternatives for getting rid of household pests. It is important to be patient and willing to try a variety of methods to evaluate which is most effective against your particular pests. Patience was the key in eliminating crickets that had invaded our home.

In our nontoxic home, we had built a subfloor under our hardwood floor, a procedure that allowed us to lay the flooring without using any glues. We never anticipated that this subfloor would also become a vacation resort for one persistent cricket.

It would not have been that bad except for the fact that this little cricket had decided to spend each and every night in the subfloor right underneath MY bed. And this cricket was obviously trying out for "Loudest Cricket of the Year Award" as it chirped and screeched all night long.

We could see the small space by the wall through which it probably had entered the subfloor, but we still could not coax the cricket out.

On the sixth sleepless night, I started thinking this nightmare was probably a pest control company's practical joke on us—the ultimate, unnerving challenge for persons determined to control pests nontoxically. What made it even more frustrating was that despite all my research and resources, I was not able to discover what might lure the little guy out.

On the ninth sleepless night, I may have even created a few Walter Mitty scenes in my head in which mysterious cans of bug spray suddenly appeared and sprayed their contents right down into that small space. Finally, a few nights later as we were going to bed, my husband spotted the cricket on the floor beside his shoe. While I would like to write that my husband simply captured the cricket and put him outside, the truth is that he jumped up, grabbed the shoe, and within seconds smashed the unsuspecting bug.

While it took us eleven days to eliminate the cricket without using chemicals, if we had used a pesticide, we might have then been exposed to harmful pesticide residues for eleven *years*.

General Approaches to Nontoxic Pest Control

Despite the number of pesticides available, humans will never completely "eliminate" insects simply because they outnumber us. Experts estimate that there may be as many as ten million different kinds of insects on the earth (the actual number of individual insects is beyond counting). However, it may be helpful to know that less than 1 percent of all insects are actually pests. Although there is no one accepted definition of a pest, the Pest Control Hotline defines a pest as any insect that has no value and can cause detrimental health in humans. Another thought to keep in mind when implementing nontoxic pest control is that whenever a new home is built the new occupants are really the intruders (not the pests) since construction automatically displaces millions of tiny animals. If a home provides a good supply of dry food and water, the "former" occupants will be encouraged to return.

General nontoxic pest control preventive measures include inspecting and repairing your home (e.g., window screens, cracks in outside walls, rusted drains, broken toilets) and modifying the landscape surrounding your home. Shrubs and flowers along the perimeter of a home serve as a wonderful entry route for pests. Laying a clear eighteen inch strip of either cement or sand around your home is a good way of creating an effective pest barricade.

In addition, remove any Algerian ivy bordering the lawn as it is a perfect habitat for black widows, rats and mice; store foods in properly sealed containers (keeping dry foods in bags and cardboard boxes is an open invitation for many pests); wipe up all spills and food immediately; deodorize your garbage cans weekly with a borax solution; eliminate clutter (e.g., old newspapers, boxes) so that pests will not have "safe" havens; rotate clothing so that all is frequently worn and cleaned (this is the best protection against fabric pests); and rearrange furniture and wall pictures periodically (this shakes up hiding pests).

If an infestation occurs, locate where the pests are entering, locate where they are finding food and water, find out what conditions are unfavorable to the pest, and make the appropriate changes.

Not all techniques are going to be equally effective for all situations. To expect to eliminate *all* the pests is not realistic. However, keep in mind that chemical insecticides cannot guarantee 100 percent success either. If you are committed to controlling pests nontoxically, you can expect very few pests *most* of the time while unquestionably enjoying a safer home *all* of the time.

Below are some specific non-toxic pest control alternatives:

Nontoxic Roach Control

Remarkably, roaches can live three months without food and thirty days without water. Since they taste their food before eating it, they learn to avoid chemically-treated surfaces. As unborn eggs, they are immune to all insecticides. They are known to nest in telephones, televisions, radios, refrigerators, electric clocks, corrugated boxes, books, draperies, old magazines and newspapers.

To prevent roaches from invading your home:

- clean the area around your water heater
- glue down any loose wallpaper behind appliances
- do not keep bags or boxes of pet food or damp dishrags under the kitchen sink
- dry up wherever moisture gathers in the bathroom
- hang rubber shower mats to dry after use (the rows of suction cups provide roaches with a custom-fitted hiding place)
- periodically inspect and clean closets, televisions, radios, and electric clocks.
- vacuum the folds of your window draperies
- throw out piles of old magazines, newspapers, boxes, and clothing
- fix dripping faucets and/or leaky toilets
- fill all cracks in walls and woodwork
- seal any gaps around water or gas pipes leading to your home
- put several inches of gravel inside the water meter vault
- move stacks of wood away from your house
- pull up ivy or other types of broad ground cover
- throw way grocery bags or corrugated cardboard boxes
- remove any leftover pet food after feeding time
- put your garbage out nightly
- carefully inspect all used furniture before purchasing

Apartment dwellers should nail window screening over shared heating vents and weatherstrip doors to any common hallway.

Recently, my housekeeper had the opportunity to sample both toxic and nontoxic pest control solutions for roaches. Despite the fact that her apartment building had been sprayed by a pest control company twice within a two-month period, her apartment was still overrun with roaches. Since she was already distressed by the apartment manager's decision to spray (she had come to learn about pesticides since working for us), she was equally distressed to still find cockroaches scurrying for cover every time she opened a cupboard or drawer.

I told her about the "drunken cockroach" trap that I had read about while researching this book. This trap consists of a rag soaked in beer. The rag attracts the roaches and, after they have become "drunk" from drinking the beer, immobilizes them for easy removal.

She tried this plan, and, to her amazement, the next morning she could not see any portion of the rag she had soaked. It was completely covered with some three hundred very drunk, immobilized roaches! She now sets this trap about once a week and tells me that she has definitely seen a remarkable improvement in her roach problem. (A pest problem can be more difficult to resolve if one lives in an apartment building since tenants cannot require their neighbors to also follow such preventive measures.)

Another nontoxic roach solution is called the "British trap." To make this trap, wrap masking tape around the outside of an empty jam jar. Fill the jar halfway with a mixture of beer, a few banana slices, and a few drops of anise extract. Next, smear a thin band of petroleum jelly just inside the rim of the jar. The food attracts the roaches, and the petroleum jelly prevents them from escaping. Twelve of these traps have been reported to net over *eight thousand* cockroaches in a three month period.

Another nontoxic way to eliminate roaches is to alter the conditions in your home. Roaches die in temperatures above 130 degrees or below 23 degrees. They thrive in temperatures of about 80 degrees.

Nontoxic Ant Control

Most of us believe that ants have no value; but, in fact, these insects enrich the soil and protect orange trees from citrus pests. Ants also prey on cockroaches and can prevent termite damage (ants will attack a wingless queen termite searching for a nest). When my four-year-old daughter learned what termites were capable of doing, she thought ants were great. She said that she would much rather have a little ant crawling by than a termite gnawing away at her home.

To prevent ant infestations, try these suggestions:

- trim all tree and shrub branches near your home (ants crawl along them to get inside a window or door crack)
- plant mint or tansy around the perimeter of your home to repel ants
- patch all window, wall, and door cracks—no matter how small
- do not over-water your yard
- immediately wipe up all spilled food
- store food in tightly closed containers

• ensure that bottles of sticky, sweet foods (e.g., jams and syrups) are wiped clean after use

When ants have entered your home, trace them back to their point of entry and seal it with petroleum, putty, or other caulking material; wash down countertops, floors, and cupboardds with equal parts of vinegar and water; sprinkle one (or all) of the following around the structure: cornmeal, red chili pepper, borax; and sprinkle borax powder inside and around trash cans. Also, locate the nest outdoors and pour boiling water or hot paraffin onto it.

If the ant nest or nests cannot be located, bait the ants by putting honey and baker's yeast in the dirt of a flower pot. When the ants arrive, destroy the new colony site with boiling water or hot paraffin. Another approach is to put just a few grains of 99 percent technical (not medicinal) boric acid and some honey in a lid from a jam jar and place it outside at night. The ants will be attracted to the honey and will take it back to their nest—but they will also take back the boric acid, which will kill the rest of the ants in the nest. While boric acid is not toxic if inhaled, it *is* toxic if swallowed by humans or other animals. Therefore, this approach should only be used when and where there is no possibility that a pet or small child might eat the honey.

I readily concede that it is quite easy to advocate nontoxic pest control when the pests are a minor problem. I have a friend who immediately stopped using pesticides when she heard what had happened to me. For several months, she eagerly shared with others that she no longer used nor needed pesticides to eliminate her kitchen ants. She would proudly inform her friends that her ant problem was effectively being controlled by simply drowning the ants in water (her own creative nontoxic solution).

But then the BIG TEST came. One morning she entered her kitchen and was greeted by hundreds of little ants—everywhere. As she faced ants in the cereal, sugar, crackers, and on the counters and pantry, she knew that this new situation required much more than a little dousing of water here and there. This was a MEGA-ANT problem.

But to her credit (and after the initial panic), she called me to find out what nontoxic alternatives she could use. Frustrated, she conveyed that although she did not want to use pesticides, the thought of sharing her kitchen with hundreds of ants was intolerable.

While talking with her, I began to realize that the ants had actually been "invited" into her home. In the past, the trees and shrubs near her home (combined with the opened boxes of food on the kitchen shelves) had always lured a few of the outside ants inside. But a recent sprinkler problem had now flooded these ants and forced them out of their outside nests. In short, the ants were simply looking for a new place to reside. I mention this because if one can identify the reason for a sudden ant invasion, then one might also be pacified and realize that the pest problem is only temporary.

After listening to the various nontoxic alternatives for getting rid of ants, my friend implemented several of the suggestions I had offered her. Three days later, she happily reported that the ant problem was under control. To some, three days might seem too long—especially after being accustomed to wiping out pests immediately. But while it may have taken my friend three days to get rid of the ants, she did not have to spend the rest of her days in haling toxic chemicals. Equally important was her firsthand proof that pesticides were not needed to eliminate ants.

Nontoxic Beetle Control

There are various types of beetles, which feed on everything from milk, cayenne pepper, legumes, corn, wheat, and rice to tobacco products, herbs, spices, grains, chocolate, dried fruits, meats, fish, vegetables, nuts, coffee beans, leather, furniture stuffing, paprika, and dog food. The cigarette beetle (which is approximately one-tenth of an inch long, reddish brown, and covered with short, fine hairs) and the drugstore beetle (which is about the same size and light brown) actually even *like* insecticides containing pyrethrum. These beetles also thrive on poisons such as acoine, belladonna, and strychnine.

To prevent beetle infestations:

• inspect food packages before purchasing them. Avoid packages that are punctured or have loose-fitting flaps.
• clean cupboards regularly
• buy staples in moderate amounts
• keep cupboards dry
• vacuum periodically to remove crumbs
• refrigerate whole grains and put a bay leaf in each opened grain container
• eliminate bird, rodent, and wasp nests near the home

Become more prudent with routine cleaning and inspection during the summer since the reproductive cycles of some beetles can be less than a week in warm temperatures.

As soon as you spot even one beetle in your home, put the infested food in a plastic bag and close it securely with a rubber band. Dispose of it in an outside garbage container in the hot sun (if possible). Put other suspect food (especially food near the infestation site) in plastic bags and quarantine. Watch for any beetles. Empty everything in the pantry and vacuum and wash all surfaces.

As is true of other pests, you can eliminate beetles by regulating the temperature in the areas where they may be found. For example, if beetles have infested raisins or other dried fruits, boil the food in hot water for one minute; the heat will kill the beetles without ruining the food. If beetles have infested your staples, you can eliminate them by heating the food in thin layers in the oven for two hours at 125 degrees or by placing the food in the freezer. These approaches may be good alternatives for individuals who do not want to throw out infested food.

Nontoxic Flea Control

When we first realized that we had to cancel our pest control service, we knew we had no choice but to seek alternative methods for controlling our never-ending flea problem. After doing a little reading, we instituted an innovative nontoxic approach. First we gave our dog large amounts of brewer's yeast to make his coat less dry and brittle. We also occasionally rubbed his coat with pennyroyal oil. In addition, we began routinely sprinkling salt onto our carpets.

In the beginning, we were skeptical. After all, even our bi-monthly professional pest control service had never been completely effective in eliminating our fleas. But our motivation to seek a nontoxic solution stemmed from the realization that we had no other choice.

With great apprehension, we awaited the grand invasion of fleas. The fact that we made it "flea-free" through the winter months did not reduce our anxiety as summer—better known as "flea fiesta" time—was just around the corner. But summer came and still nothing happened. Not one flea. Five months passed. Six months. Seven months. Then, finally, after eight flea-free months we ultimately concluded that we were, in fact, successfully deterring the pests non-chemically. More impressive was the fact that with toxic chemicals we never had even enjoyed two flea-free months.

After we read further into the literature on chemical-free alternatives, we began to understand part of our success. Without question, the vitamin B in the brewer's yeast *had* changed our dog's coat from dry and brittle to silky and shiny. This new coat, it turns out, was not as inviting to fleas. The pennyroyal repelled the fleas (and anything else that did not like the smell of peppermint), and the salt in the carpet created a dehydrated environment in which fleas cannot thrive. (Note: Pennyroyal has been associated with spontaneous abortions and should not be used around pregnant women or pets.)

Yet, fleas can be difficult to control since they can lay six hundred eggs a month and can remain in the pupa stage (in a cocoon) from one week to one year, not coming out until they sense the right conditions (e.g., warmth, humidity, carbon dioxide from a nearby host, etc.).

The most obvious way to keep fleas out of the home is to keep pets outside. But I know this is unacceptable to many pet lovers. Other nontoxic ways to help curb fleas include:

- combing your pet everyday with a flea comb (in warm weather)
- feeding your dog brewer's yeast (use twenty-five milligrams per ten pounds of animal weight)
- using herbal or fatty acid flea shampoos
- rubbing herbal repellents (e.g., citronella, tea tree oil, eucalyptus oil) into your pet's fur

In addition, occasionally apply a citrus oil to your pet's fur while brushing its coat. To make the oil, cover four cut lemons with water in a saucepan. Boil, and then simmer forty-five minutes. Cool and strain the liquid. Some pets may need to be dusted liberally with pyrethrum powder to kill and control fleas in between shampoos. Pyrethrum is a nontoxic pesticide that works by drying out the protective coating of hard shelled pests; in addition to directly applying it on the pet, it can also be sprinkled on carpet and outside areas.

A pet's diet also plays a role. I used to laugh at pet owners who only bought "high quality" pet food, but it turns out that commercial pet foods actually intensify flea infestation, because many of them contain meat by-products. In contrast, high quality pet foods found in health food stores usually use only US grade A meat ingredients with lots of yeast, garlic, and herbs. It seems that a strong, healthy pet does not attract fleas as easily.

If fleas have infested your home, vacuum frequently (and put the vacuum bag in the freezer to kill the fleas). High temperatures will also kill fleas, so heat your home to 122 degrees for several hours (when you and your pets will not be home). You can also sprinkle a dehydrating agent, such as unprocessed Diatomeceous Earth (not the kind used for pools), which works in the same way as pyrethrum powder, on your carpet, deck, and lawn. Applying this to the outside will reduce the number of fleas your pet comes in contact with outside each day.

Another innovative way to kill fleas is referred to as "flea suicide." To use this approach, fill a shallow dish with detergent and water, set a flash-light over the dish, and leave it near a flea infestation site. Leave the light on at night. This set-up will attract the fleas so that they will jump into the wa-ter and drown. One person reported that he was able to catch over five hun-dred fleas in just three days with this method.

Nontoxic Silverfish Control

Silverfish, insects with fish-like bodies that live in damp places and books, may be entering a home via the wallboard or green lumber or through flowers near the home's foundation. Silverfish love wood shavings, sawdust, wallpaper paste, the sizing on paper, cereals, dead insects, linen, cotton, silk, and bookbinding glue. They like to hide and lay their eggs in wall cracks and behind baseboards.

Because silverfish thrive on the mulch in flower beds, it is necessary to relocate flowers away from the foundation of the home. Other preventive measures include routinely cleaning bookcases and shaking out books, re-pairing plumbing leaks, and periodically checking the lining and outer fab-ric of all lined draperies.

If silverfish are discovered in the home , you can eliminate them with a simple trap. Cover the outside of a small glass jar with masking tape and place a small amount of wheat flour inside. Set the trap in a corner. The sil-verfish will crawl up the tape and fall into the jar; however, the slippery in-terior walls of the jar will prevent them from climbing out.

Nontoxic Termite Control

Termites are divided into two major groups: drywood (living above the earth) and subterranean (living below the earth). Drywood termites nest in the wood they eat, have relatively small colonies, and can go without mois-ture for long periods of time. Subterranean termites nest in the ground, but feed above it by tunneling up and building flattened shelter tubes. They like homes with central heating. They do not like to be shaken, however, and thus avoid such objects as musical instruments, railroad ties, or anything else that vibrates. As many as a quarter of a million termites can be found in a single subterranean colony.

A mass of tiny wings scattered on the ground is an early sign of termite infestation. This is because termites shed their wings after mating; they then burrow into wood and lay their eggs. Signs of termite infestation include the appearance of shelter tubes, particles of earth and wood cemented together with a glue-like secretion; dark or blistered areas of wood flooring; and/or six-sided fecal pellets (considered the calling card of drywood termites).

To prevent termite infestation, place a sand barrier around your home as termites cannot burrow through sand. Make sure that basement air vents are fully exposed and not overgrown with shrubbery, avoid sprinkling stucco or wood siding when watering, repair any faulty plumbing, and check that downspouts and gutters carry water away from the house.

When termites are already in the home, a natural predator such as ants can be used to eliminate them. For example, the dirt tubes which the termites create to climb on top of edible surfaces can be broken and ants can be inserted. The ants will seek out and destroy the termites. Predator nematodes can also be used. Other nontoxic approaches include setting external corrugated cardboard traps (termites prefer corrugated cardboard to wood), altering the temperature in the house (some major pest control companies now offer liquid nitrogen as an alternative to chemical fumigation), and employing a company that uses an electrogun to eliminate termites (which kills termites with electric volts).

Nontoxic Treatment for Head Lice

As a teacher, I once received a grant to have my students simulate Southeast Asia. On the day of the big event, a shy Hmong student arrived at school with a suitcase carrying the traditional Hmong native dress that I had happily agreed to wear. However, I had forgotten about the headgear that went with this native apparel. After my student and her grandmother finished wrapping the many layers of the dress around me, they then brought out the turban. I knew that this incredibly embroidered outfit had been passed down for generations. As I looked at what I was wearing and at the turban, I couldn't help but ask, "Gee, how do you wash all this?" My student and her grandmother smiled and shook their heads as they told me, "No, no—you do not wash this [ceremonial] dress."

Upon hearing that, I immediately thought of LICE. But since I could not deny the incredible pride on my student's face as she shared her native ceremonial dress with me, I took a big gulp and put on the turban.

But, the first time my scalp itched the next day, I was convinced that I had lice. Even though there was no real evidence, I decided to be on the safe side. I went out and bought some lice shampoo. Only now I know that what I did was not "on the safe side" at all since I was applying pesticides to my head. Back then I knew nothing about the dangers associated with pesticide shampoo, and I certainly didn't know of any nontoxic ways to get rid of lice.

However, I now know that the following nontoxic suggestions will eliminate head lice without jeopardizing the health of either you or your child.

The following nontoxic steps should be taken for the treatment of home and personal articles:

1. Using *hot* water, machine wash all clothing and bed linen which has come in contact with the infested person within the past three days.

2. Carefully vacuum all rugs and upholstered furniture, mattresses, stuffed animals, etc., to pick up any living lice or nits that may have attached themselves to them.

For treating the individual, it is important to note that while the National Pediculosis Association (NPA) specifically discourages the use of shampoos with the chemical lindane, the association also points out that *all* lice treatments on the market today are pesticides. While some of these pesticides, such as pyrethrin, might be considered less toxic than lindane, there still remains the problem of the petroleum distillates (which are not usually identified) that are included in the pesticide formulas. Keep in mind that whatever chemical is applied, it is going to be easily absorbed into the bloodstream since the scalp is so porous. The following nontoxic approach for individuals is recommended:

1. Wet the hair thoroughly with warm water and apply a fatty acid based shampoo (see Appendix 2). Cover the entire head and all of the hair.

2. Rinse with warm water and repeat the process described in step one; however, this time leave suds on the hair.

3. Tie a towel around the soapy hair and leave on for approximately thirty minutes.

4. Remove towel and comb hair first with a regular comb and then with a nit-removing comb. If the hair begins to dry during the process, dampen it slightly with water. It may take as long as two hours to remove all the nits.

5. Wash the hair for a third time. Rinse and dry.

6. Inspect the hair and scalp for any lice that you may have missed.

7. Check hair again in seven to ten days for any lice nits that you may have missed which have subsequently hatched.

Nontoxic Pest Control Companies

One reason nontoxic pest control companies may continue to be rare might stem from the public's misguided notion of what pest control actually is. Since I began implementing nontoxic approaches, I now realize that pest control companies have nothing to do with controlling pests—despite the fact that all their trucks say **PEST CONTROL**. Rather, pest control companies just come into your house and spray chemicals. I now know that true pest control does not involve spraying according to some pre-established schedule. Instead, effective pest control focuses on identifying the source of the problem and utilizing preventive measures.

However, before they agree to sign a contract, typical pest control company customers want to know the cost and the number of times their school, business, and/or home will be serviced. An authentic nontoxic company cannot realistically follow this format. When using a nontoxic approach, "nature" is very much involved. Even the most competent entomologist cannot make Mother Nature comply with a pre-established schedule. Yet, since the goal of nontoxic pest control companies is to *control* pests rather than expose you and your family to repeated exterminations, the overall cost for a nontoxic pest control service will ultimately be significantly less.

If you cannot locate a nontoxic service in your area, employ a landscape architect who focuses on natural approaches to the land. You can also continually call existing pest control companies to ask if any nontoxic services are available. Some established pest control companies are already offering nontoxic treatments for termites. If companies get enough calls for a service they are more likely to offer it in the future. After all, business is business.

NONTOXIC SCHOOL GROUND MAINTENANCE

In direct contrast to schools that overuse and/or are dependent on toxic chemicals, some individual school districts have adopted programs that either greatly reduce or eliminate pesticide applications on school grounds. These programs emphasize preventive maintenance, design changes, systemic monitoring, and the use of nontoxic or least toxic approaches for treatment. Such programs can be very cost effective. For example, in Eugene, Oregon, implementation of an Integrated Pest Management program cut the district's annual pesticide bill by more than two-thirds.[12]

To assist schools in adopting new pest control policies, the Northwest

Coalition for Alternatives to Pesticides (NCAP) has developed an eighty-six page packet entitled "Planning for Non-Chemical School Ground Maintenance." The packet describes both the policy and the strategic steps necessary for the successful adoption of a less toxic school ground maintenance plan.

In the interim, parents can request that their child's school complete both the School Pesticide Survey (Appendix 3) and the School Toxicology Information Sheet (Appendix 4) so parents can begin to assess the chemicals to which their children are exposed at school. If the school district is not able to supply adequate information about the chemicals it uses, parents can ask the EPA to provide the following information: whether or not the EPA has completed a "registration standard" for the product (if so, request a copy); whether or not there is missing or falsified data supporting the product's registration; whether or not the chemicals are one the EPA's list for special review; and whether or not the product has ever been either voluntarily or involuntarily canceled and why. If necessary, parents can file a Freedom of Information Act to obtain all health and environmental effects studies done on the product in question.

Parents can also ask to be notified when chemicals are going to be used on the school grounds and to be given the name of the specific chemical being applied. If school nurses also had this information, they could determine if there was an increase in the number of students complaining of asthma or other health related problems.

REDUCING EXPOSURES TO PESTICIDE APPLICATIONS

I would like to have omitted this section simply because I want to believe that if you have reached this point, you are no longer considering using pesticides at all. But since I know that I am not on Fantasy Island, I feel obligated to include suggestions on how to reduce pesticide exposures if you are *still* going to use pesticides in your home. These suggestions include:

- mix only the amount of pesticide needed to solve the current problem
- never store mixed pesticides
- refrain from spraying on windy or foggy days
- avoid exposing bees as they are extremely sensitive to various pesticides and will likely sting everything in sight
- do not smoke or stand near someone who is smoking while spraying pesticides

- keep children away from areas being sprayed
- wash your clothing and yourself immediately following the application of pesticides

PROPOSED PESTICIDE REFORMS

The following suggestion for reform would greatly reduce the current loopholes in pesticide legislation and policy. Your awareness of these reforms and your involvement in getting them implemented can play a major role in ridding toxins from our environment.

Proposed Registration Laws

- The EPA would be required to refuse to register any pesticide for which complete data has not been submitted.
- Conditional registrations would not be permitted.
- The EPA would be able to ban or suspend pesticides whose registration was based on invalid testing.
- The EPA would be able to deny registration solely on the basis of human health risks.
- Manufacturers would be required to prove that their product is effective prior to registration.

Proposed Pesticide Laws

- Pesticide product labels would be required to include *all* ingredients.
- Reprisals for "outspoken" employees (acting within the law) would be a federal offense.
- The EPA would be required to set air and surface pesticide standards for the home.
- Commercial applicators would be required to file annual reports with the EPA regarding the time, place, quantities, and mixtures of pesticides applied.

Letters from a large number of citizens can be very influential in changing government policy. Write letters to your senators and congresspersons at the addresses below.

The Honorable (name of senator)
U.S. Senate
Washington, D.C. 20510

The Honorable (name of representative)
U S. House of Representatives
Washington, D.C. 20515

Topics for letters:

A) Request that Section 17 of the Federal Insecticide, Rodenticide and Fungicide Act (FIRFA) be amended to make it illegal to export banned or unregistered pesticides.

B) Request that "set tolerance" levels be re-calculated.

C) Request that testing include risks from total exposures to pesticides in food, drinking water, and gardens, in both household and community applications.

D) Request that testing evaluate the risks for when toxic chemicals are combined.

E) Request that inert ingredients be tested.

F) Request that testing evaluate neurological damage other than paralysis and death that can result from pesticide use, such as possible effects on memory, behavior, learning, and motor control.

G) Request that pesticides that cannot be detected by routine methods be prohibited. Without this type of law, it is virtually impossible for the FDA to enforce EPA guidelines.

You can also write the World Bank and request that it end its present policy of only financing chemically-dependent agriculture in third world countries.

The World Bank
1818 H Street NW
Washington, D.C. 20433

IN THE FUTURE

Two years ago, the only thing I knew about pesticides was that my pest control service was always a little late. Fortunately, despite my own past ignorance, many groups and individuals have been earnestly working for a long time to promote consumer awareness and to change existing practices.

For example, as a result of public pressure, Uniroyal finally decided to pull the chemical Alar off the market. In spite of dark predictions of gloom, this year's domestic apple crop did not suffer without Alar. In fact, the crop was actually *10 percent larger than in 1988.*[13]

The town of Wauconda, Illinois, took a different kind of positive action. The town enacted an ordinance which required lawn companies to post warning signs during and after pesticide applications. However, not surprisingly, a major pesticide company, ChemLawn, sued the town mayor and trustees claiming that the town did not have the power to make such an ordinance.

The court initially ruled in the company's favor, stating that the local ordinance was not necessary since state legislation provided adequate protection. That decision has since been overturned. This conflict between small town and major chemical company may well end up in the Supreme Court. However, while Wauconda's battle continues, other places across the country have followed their lead. In several states, signs are posted in many public places indicating when the area is sprayed and what chemicals are used.

ChemLawn also became the center of attention in the state of New York when State Attorney General Robert Abrams won a lawsuit against the company for advertising that its products are "practically nontoxic" and "do not present a health risk."

And in Oregon, the State Department of Human Resources sent suggested guidelines for pesticide use to all school superintendents. This action was the result of several incidents in which both children and staff became ill following the application of pesticides on school grounds.

Numerous non-profit groups of concerned citizens have also been formed at the international, national, state, and local levels. One project of the international organization Greenpeace is to call upon all industrialized countries to prohibit the export of banned, severely restricted, or unregistered pesticides.

Mothers and Others for a Livable Planet was recently established to give a unified voice to families concerned about pesticides in food. A sampling of other major organizations working on pesticide issues includes: Americans for Safe Food, the National Coalition Against the Misuse of Pesticides, the Natural Resource Defense Council, and the Northwest Coalition for Alternatives to Pesticides. Each group is motivated by a strong, shared belief that current pesticide practices, policies, and laws need to be carefully reconsidered and changed.

Recently, I read the testimony an eleven-year-old boy gave before a senate committee. This boy has such severe reactions to pesticides that he is unable to visit parks, public schools, or, in short, almost any other place where you are likely to find an eleven-year-old. In fact, after he gave his testimony he had to be led from the room and treated with oxygen because he suffered a severe reaction to the clothing of the next speaker—a member of the pest control industry.

In his testimony, this young boy expressed his sorrow, his anger, and his hopelessness about the persistence of pesticides in our world. He is afraid that the continued use of pesticides will force him to abandon his dream of ever playing on a baseball team since he will never be able to get near a field.

But I would like him to hold on to that dream. I believe that as more and more people start to truly understand how dangerous pesticides are they will be motivated to seek nontoxic alternatives for controlling pests. My dream for this little boy is that one day his mother will watch her son eagerly approach the plate as she proudly shouts from the stands, "Hit a home run, slugger! Hit a home run!"

CHECKLIST FOR SUGGESTED CHANGES
AND COMMITMENTS

☐ Petition your local grocery store to carry organically grown food. Meet with the produce manager, write the corporate management, and supply the store with a list of organic growers. In the interim, request that your supermarket label the origin of all produce and buy only domestically grown food that is in season.

☐ Eat only organically grown food.

☐ Use only nontoxic alternatives, both indoors and outdoors, for eliminating pests.

☐ Call the maintenance department of your local city parks to inquire about spraying schedules so you can avoid the parks on these days. However, keep in mind, that as with home lawn care applications, most pesticides are designed to have lasting effects. Pesticide residues may still linger into the next day, week, or even the next month.

☐ Request information from your school district concerning when and how often chemicals are applied on school grounds, and what kind of testing has been submitted to the EPA for these chemicals.

☐ Organize a group to work with the PTA and/or school district personnel to have an integrated pest control program (as opposed to a traditional program of routine sprayings and applications) implemented at your child's school. The same group can also work to encourage local parks to implement integrated pest control.

☐ Organize neighborhood cooperation for posting signs to warn families when front lawns have been recently treated with chemicals— especially during the summer when children tend to run barefoot and can easily come in direct contact with pesticide residues.

☐ Write letters to your senators and congresspersons requesting legislation changes.

☐ Support, join, and/or become involved in a non-profit group working to ensure safe usage, reduction, and/or elimination of pesticides (see Appendix 2).

Quiz 3—A Pretest on Daily Toxins

1. Chemicals can enter your body through ingestion and
_____.
     A) skin absorption
     B) nose and/or mouth inhalation
     C) all of the above

2. Approximately _____ percent of labels on household items on the market today have some type of error (e.g., incorrect first aid information, omission that a product contains a poison).[1]
     A) 10 percent
     B) 34 percent
     C) 85 percent

3. A study of the toxic effects of formaldehyde revealed that _____ persons is sensitive to this chemical.
     A) one in twenty
     B) one in ten
     C) one in five

4. The fact that a fabric has been treated with formaldehyde resins is
_____.
     A) required by law to be noted on the label
     B) required by law to be noted on the label of permanent press clothing only
     C) not required by law to be noted on any clothing label

5. Perchloroethylene, a solvent that can cause cancer, liver damage, depression of the central nervous system, light-headedness, dizziness, insomnia, loss of appetite, and disorientation, is used extensively by the _____ industry.
     A) dry cleaning
     B) auto
     C) food

6. Cleaning product manufacturers are required by law to
_____.
     A) inform consumers of any type of hazards associated with their products
     B) print on label all ingredients used to make the product
     C) neither A nor B

7. Individuals can be exposed daily to toxic chemicals, such as toluene, benzene, and naphtha, that are released from solvent based
_____.

    A) adhesives and paints
    B) waxes and cleaners
    C) upholstery and plastic
    D) all of the above

8. The total toxic contamination load of newer homes is primarily due to
_____.

    A) the prevalence of new synthetic materials and energy-efficient construction
    B) the use of lead paint

Answers to Daily Toxins Quiz

1. C The effects of inhaled and/or swallowed toxic substances are usually well-known; however, skin absorption is frequently overlooked. For example, many consumers insist on buying purified water to drink, yet think nothing of taking a bath in the toxic water they wouldn't drink. Between 50 and 60 percent of the absorption of contaminants from tap water occurs through the skin.

2. C Labels frequently contain incorrect information concerning the danger of a product. Additionally, according to Poison Control Centers, the first aid information printed on product labels (e.g., what to do if the product is accidentally ingested) is often incorrect and could actually cause more harm if followed.

3. C Formaldehyde is found in countless products. It is most often used in resin glues, plastics, and foam. Additionally, it is commonly used as a preservative, fungicide, and stabilizer and is produced by combustion (e.g., cigarette smoke, natural gas). Some symptoms of formaldehyde sensitivity include respiratory irritation, headaches, dizziness, heart palpitations, severe depression, shortness of breath, and swelling of the throat.

4. C While manufacturers are not required by law to indicate the use of formaldehyde resins on clothing, words such as "crease resistant," "permanent press," "no-iron," or "water-repellant" on a label clearly indicate its use. In general, it can be assumed that virtually all polyester/cotton blend fabrics have formaldehyde finishes. It should also be noted that polyester/cotton bed linens will typically have an even heavier formaldehyde finish since they must stand up to weekly laundering.

5. A   Dry cleaned garments are often returned to customers before the chemicals used in the cleaning process have completely evaporated. Since inhaling perchloroethylene (and other chemicals used in dry cleaning) can be very dangerous, it is advisable to air out all dry cleaned items in a well-ventilated area for at least a few days prior to wearing.

6. C   While manufacturers are required to print the word "caution" or "warning" on the labels of products that contain known hazardous substance(s), they don't have to print the name of the substance. Additionally, there is no law that requires cleaning manufacturers to warn consumers against possible hazards associated with their product. For example, the American Lung Association warns people not to use aerosol sprays since aerosol mist can aggravate existing lung conditions. Yet aerosol spray manufacturers do not mention this on their product labels.

7. D   These dangerous chemicals are commonly used in items that consumers are exposed to daily. They can cause dizziness, disorientation, fatigue, muscle weakness, and irritation of the skin and lungs. Some are carcinogenic or have been known to cause kidney or liver damage. Most are soluble in fatty tissue and are readily absorbed and subsequently stored in some bodies.

8. A   Today, indoor air contaminants are more likely to build up in newer, energy-efficient buildings and homes because they have poorer ventilation. In addition, the use of chemicals in building materials and fabrics has increased more than fivefold over the past twenty years.

CHAPTER THREE

Toxins—At Home, In the Neighborhood

We simply could not put off cleaning the oven any longer. The black, baked-on remnants from six months worth of dinners just had to go. However, the thought of oven-cleaner fumes permeating the house horrified me. Even before my new chemical sensitivities, odors emitted by oven cleaners (though I still used various products) always seemed offensive and rather intrusive to me since they baked right along with (or into?) my next few casseroles.

I now know that oven cleaners contain petroleum distillates, which are central nervous depressants; methylene chloride, a chlorinated hydrocarbon stored in the fatty tissue which is toxic to the liver and kidneys; lye, a corrosive poison; and other toxic chemicals. Therefore, we knew that we could not even consider using a commercial oven cleaner. So, we consulted Debra Dadd's book *Nontoxic and Natural* to see what she recommended for cleaning ovens.

I should note here that we did this when nontoxic alternatives were very new to us, and we were still a little skeptical of them. We were, after all, probably talking about the dirtiest oven of the year.

As my husband read the suggestions in the book, he shook his head and commented with undeniable sarcasm, "Right, this is really going to work."

However, with these nontoxic alternatives as our only options, my husband finally decided to try the baking soda and water technique. My husband was convinced that none of the book's suggestions would ever work, but this idea seemed to him the best since it was most likely to fail in the shortest amount of time.

Following the book's suggestions, he first soaked the oven walls with water. Then, he applied a generous amount of the baking soda to the sides of the oven. After allowing the baking soda to sit for a short period of time, he took his sponge and began to wipe off the baking soda.

When my husband would later tell people what happened next, his voice would rise about ten octaves as he would exclaim, "The stuff just wiped off! Everything! Every piece of caked-on crud just slid right off! It was AMAZ-ING!" I would tease him that his enthusiastic testimonial was far more convincing than any T.V. commercial.

After this success with a nontoxic cleaning alternative, we began substituting nontoxic products for toxic ones for almost everything we used. We first went through all the medicine cabinets and bathroom drawers, throwing out toxic products. Next, we cleared out all the toxic products from the laundry room, the kitchen, and the garage. This included everything from unquestionably toxic items such as drain cleaners and bleaches to less obviously toxic ones such as commercial shampoos and deodorants. It was surprising just how much there was. Even more incredible was the small number of items that were needed to replace all the specialized products (furniture polish, tile cleaner, floor cleaner, etc.) that we had previously thought we needed.

Later, we would continue to make changes on a larger scale when we moved into our new "pesticide-free" home. But, undeniably, our transition from a toxic to a nontoxic lifestyle began in our old home. Clearly, we were motivated to make the changes because of my health. But, to our pleasant surprise, we found that nontoxic living is both easy and fun.

I readily concede that it is unsettling to think that one's home may be filled with toxins. I remember how long it took me to accept that every room and just about everything in my home was, in fact, contributing to creating a toxic environment. But, on the other hand, to ignore the possibility that one's home may be filled with toxic substances may ultimately result in the ill health of one or more family members.

It is often difficult to tell just by a home's appearance whether or not it is toxic. My old home did not suggest any kind of doom. In fact, it was a very desirable residence in a fashionable neighborhood. People would often praise its interior design, fantastic views, and large redwood deck. Yet, our *beautiful* home was not a *safe* home. In fact, the word "pretty," often used to describe our home, turned out to mean "pretty deadly" for us.

"Pretty deadly," unfortunately, may describe too many homes. In one five-year study, the EPA found that a number of homes had chemical levels that were seventy times higher inside the homes than outside. Additionally, a report by the Consumer Product Safety Commission on chemicals commonly found in homes identified 150 which have been linked to allergies, birth defects, cancer, and psychological abnormalities.[2] While outdoor pollution and air quality is at least monitored, no one monitors the levels of pollutants or the quality of the air *inside* a home. And, chances are, most individuals spend twelve to twenty hours a day in this unmonitored environment.

This chapter looks at possible sources of toxins in a typical home and offers practical suggestions for using nontoxic alternatives. While the first part of the chapter may be shocking and/or depressing (after all, who likes to think of his or her home as poisonous), I hope the reader will be challenged to make some of the changes described in the second half. Hopefully, after finishing the chapter, the reader will realize that "home" can still be "where the heart is"—it just doesn't have to also be where the toxins are.

THE PROBLEMS

TOXINS IN THE HOME

The Ongoing Outgassing

The primary problem with many materials found in a home is that even items that appear to be solid continually outgas invisible toxic vapors. For example, although a piece of furniture appears to be a solid mass, the chemicals in it are not permanently bound within the structure of the material. Rather, the chemicals are slowly and continually released into the air.

Formaldehyde is a good example of a common vapor that is outgassed in many homes. Formaldehyde is often used because it is inexpensive; it acts as an effective preservative, fungicide, and stabilizer; and it makes fabric wrinkle-free or fireproof. It appears in many building and furnishing materials (e.g., particle board, chip board, plywood, carpets, pads, construction adhesives, paints, furniture, upholstery foam, plaster, and fabrics) as well as in other products (e.g., paper goods, cosmetics, toothpaste). It is also found in homes because it is produced by the burning of gas, oil, wood, and tobacco.

Many people are already aware of the adverse health effects of formaldehyde. When the price of heating fuel skyrocketed in the mid-1970s, UFFI (urea formaldehyde foam insulation) was sprayed into the walls of many homes. In many cases, more than half of the occupants of the homes thus sprayed experienced adverse health effects due to the formaldehyde continually outgassing. As a result, UFFI was banned, and a program was initiated to remove it from homes in which it had been applied.

Yet formaldehyde is still prevalent in homes via other products, furnishings, and building materials despite the UFFI incident and the fact that in 1981 the National Institute for Occupational Safety and Health (NIOSH) stated that formaldehyde should be handled carefully because it is a potential human carcinogen (causing cancer). It is also suspected of being a teratogen (causing birth defects) and a mutagen (causing genetic damage).

Some other primary concerns with exposure to formaldehyde are that it can irritate the respiratory system, cause skin reactions, and trigger heart palpitations. Exposure to formaldehyde has also been shown to cause headaches, depression, dizziness, and loss of sleep. It can also aggravate coughs and colds or trigger asthma.

One of the most disturbing effects of formaldehyde is that after an initial exposure, such as from a new carpet, subsequent exposures to even lower concentrations of formaldehyde might trigger symptoms in the future. This is because the person has now become "sensitized" to formaldehyde. Sometimes even the most minute exposure can cause symptoms in a sensitized person. Besides formaldehyde, people can also become sensitized to other chemicals that are outgassed.

Although we cannot actually see chemicals outgassing, most of us have probably associated specific "smells" with new products and buildings. However, we probably did not know that these odors were from outgassing chemicals or that inhaling these vapors could be harmful. Also keep in mind that the absence of odor does not mean that the outgassing has stopped since this process continues long past our ability to smell it.

With a brief, general understanding of the outgassing process, we can begin to understand how homes may have significantly high levels of indoor pollutants. We can also begin to understand how many people may have become ill just from living in their house.

Synthetic, Upholstered Furniture

Formaldehyde is so prevalent in furniture that in one study the level of formaldehyde in an empty house tripled when the furniture was brought in. For example, dresser drawer fronts and furniture tops made from medium density fiberboard are considered significant sources of formaldehyde.

Other materials used in furniture construction are also known to cause adverse health affects. The stuffing in upholstered furniture can contain polyurethane foam, styrene foam chips, or foamed rubber, all of which are considered hazardous contaminants. Furniture can also be covered with acetate, nylon, or polyester fibers, which continually outgas harmful vapors. The woodwork of furniture may have been treated with a wood preservative called pentachlorophenol or a related substance called creosote. Both of these chemicals, which are brushed on wood to prevent decay and to repel insects, have been known to cause birth defects.

Another piece of furniture that is a potential toxic hazard is the bed. Beds are of significant concern because of the amount of time people spend in them. The bed is supposed to be the place where our bodies rest and detox naturally throughout the night. Yet, most people are probably sleeping on mattresses made of polyester, polyurethane, and flame retardants. All of these substances continually outgas chemicals.

The story of a woman I recently met underscores just how dramatically a toxic bed can affect one's health. This woman suffered symptoms that were very similar to what I had experienced the year before. However, she had not yet figured out that it was the repeated exposures to chemicals that were making her sick. She told me her condition had deteriorated rapidly during the last six months. Ironically, six months earlier her husband had bought her a new bed, since she spent so much time resting. It had never occurred to either of them that the new bed might actually be aggravating her condition. After she realized that chemicals were responsible for her ill-health, she immediately got rid of her new bed and began making other nontoxic changes.

Carpet

When a fellow patient at the detox clinic told me that I would have to rip out all the carpet in my house since it was obviously contributing to my overall ill health, I remember looking at her as if she were nuts (or maybe detoxing a little too much that day) and saying something like, "You really think I'm going to rip out 2,400 square feet of plush carpet that is less than three years old?" Back then, I didn't understand why carpeting is so harmful. I do now. If you love wall-to-wall carpet, you might want to skip this section because other than providing warmth and a sound barrier, there is nothing good about carpet—new or old.

Most new carpet is made from synthetic fibers which have been derived from petroleum. During the manufacturing process, crude oil is transformed into a polymer, spun into fibers, and attached to a backing. These chemical fibers are often treated with additional chemicals to make the carpet fire- or stain-resistant. Likewise, the carpet may have been treated with a fungicide or pesticide.

The following chemicals may be outgassed from carpet: benzene and formaldehyde, both suspected of causing cancer; methacrylate; tetrachloroethylene; toluene, which affects the central nervous system; and xylene, which can cause nausea and headaches. In addition, carpet pads, carpet backing, and carpet glues also outgas toxic vapors. NASA is so concerned about the outgassing of synthetic materials that it tests everything going into a spacecraft for toxicity. Not surprisingly, synthetic carpet will never see the moon.

One-hundred percent cotton or wool carpet is not necessarily chemical-free either. The carpet may have been treated with a potentially toxic dye or may have been chemically mothproofed.

The Consumer Product and Safety Commission in Washington, D.C., has printed signs warning consumers of the possible adverse health effects that can result from the installation of new carpet. The sign in my doctor's office lists burning of eyes, nose, and/or sinus cavities and breathing difficulties as commonly reported symptoms. The sign also includes a toll-free phone number for people to call if they think they have been affected by new carpet.

I have to admit I was a little surprised to see such a warning posted in my doctor's office. I could not help but wonder how many people must have already been made sick by new carpet to warrant a department of the federal government to post signs and create a hotline to address the problem.

Since carpet chemicals have been designed to be water insoluble, neither shampooing nor steaming will reduce the outgassing of toxic vapors from new carpets. In fact, the ingredients of carpet shampoo itself may be extremely toxic. For example, sodium dodecylsulfate, a common ingredient found in many carpet shampoos, is known to cause eye and skin irritations, severe respiratory distress, and headaches.

Despite all the problems with new carpet, old carpet is actually no better. Once old carpet starts to decompose, it begins to release dust. The dust irritates the respiratory tract. The dust is also pulled through the duct work of a home's heating system, and as the synthetic materials within the dust burn, they give off toxic vapors.

Old carpet is a haven for bacteria, molds, yeast, and other microorganisms. We are not just talking about a few microorganisms here and there. Scientific studies have measured ten *million* microorganisms in a square foot of carpet. Recently, my family and I watched a television program that showed some of the microorganisms found in a carpet. After seeing all those hidden bugs, my youngest daughter emphatically declared, "I sure don't want carpet in my house!"

These microorganisms flourish in humid environments, such as carpeted kitchens, bathrooms, and laundry rooms. In fact, a microorganism's dream resort is created when carpet is laid directly on a cement slab because moisture can then continually come up through the ground.

Also, forget the vacuum cleaner as a way to eliminate the microorganisms in your carpet. Routine vacuuming actually *increases* the number of microorganisms in your carpet by pulling them up from the padding to the higher layers of the carpet.

Paint and Wallpaper

Even those people who are not chemically sensitive cannot deny that a newly painted room has a distinctive smell. However, most people probably do not think about what it is they are smelling. A study done at Johns Hopkins University revealed that over 300 toxic chemicals and 150 carcinogens may be present in paint.

When paint is applied, volatile organic compounds (which are extracted from petroleum oil and gas or are produced synthetically) can reach very high concentrations—greater than 100 parts per million (ppm). This is alarming because some chemicals found in paint (benzene, for example) are considered toxic at levels over 1 ppm.

Consumers can currently choose from a variety of commercial paints. However, each kind of paint presents a problem. For example, all types of latex paint contain acrylics and synthetic rubber, as well as mold retardants and preservatives (biocides), which may or may not be listed on the label. Biocides are used as part of the paint's basic ingredients but are also added in the final stages of manufacturing to prolong the paint's shelf life.

Recently, mercury in paints has made headlines. On June 29, 1990, the EPA banned the use of mercury in indoor paints after a child whose home was painted with paint containing 930 ppm mercury (THREE TIMES the legal level of 300 ppm) was severely poisoned. Following negotiations, the EPA and paint companies agreed that the manufacturing of interior paint containing mercury would be unlawful as of August 1990. However, this law does not apply to adhesives, spackling, or joint compounds, all of which also contain mercury.

Companies that manufacture paint containing mercury are now required to label the paint "for outdoor use only." The EPA is now assessing what risks *exterior* paints with mercury pose to painters and residents.

Oil-based paints provide a better vapor-proof finish than do latex paints, but they are very toxic and may take months to become completely odorless because they contain petroleum solvents which outgas very slowly.

Instead of paint, some chose to cover their walls with wallpaper. While all wallpaper presents problems, vinyl and self-stick wallpaper are considered the most toxic because of the chemicals they outgas. Wallpaper also often contains anti-insect and/or anti-mold chemicals that can cause serious health problems. For example, wallpaper can be contaminated with diazinon, dursban, and heptachlor. Wallpaper paste also outgasses an array of chemicals.

Cabinets and Closets

Most cabinets constructed since the 1970s contain at least some particle board (usually for the interior shelves), primarily because it is so inexpensive. However, particle board is an infamous source of formaldehyde (the problems of which have already been discussed).

The clothes hanging in a typical closet are another potential source of outgassing chemicals since clothing is often made of nylon, acrylic, and polyester. According to NASA research, polyester outgasses more than any other synthetic material. However, all synthetic clothing outgasses since the fibers of such clothing are actually very soft thermoplastics made from petrochemicals that never stop vaporizing. Other clothing in your closet may be giving off vapors from commercial mothproofing or from trichloroethylene, a chemical used in the dry cleaning process.

I think that had I not become so ill two years ago, I might have a difficult time believing that *my clothes* could be harming me. Yet, it was clothing that became my first clue that I had chemical sensitivities. As the reader may recall, after a month on the Candida treatment my condition had improved significantly. But, there were still days when I regressed to the same condition I had been in eight months earlier. Christmas Day was one of those days.

I woke up that morning feeling as well as I had thus progressed. I happily went downstairs to watch my children open their presents. As they tried on their new dresses and nightgowns, and I tried on a new blouse, I started becoming quite ill. At that time, I did not know that formaldehyde is often in clothing.

After opening the gifts, I could barely get dressed to go to my in-laws for Christmas dinner. Once there, as everyone opened more presents and tried on more new clothing, I became even sicker. In fact, I had trouble sitting up for more than a few seconds.

When I felt better the next day, I became convinced that there must have been something unusual about Christmas Day that had prompted my relapse. We began to suspect the new clothes. It was this experience that first led us to discover that formaldehyde is not just in biology labs and funeral homes.

Stoves and Microwaves

There have actually been case studies of women who complain of headaches and fatigue every time they enter their kitchens. As it turns out, these women are not just trying to get out of cooking dinner; they are reacting to one or more of the many toxic substances and vapors that can be found in the average American kitchen.

According to researchers at California's Lawrence Berkeley Lab, a gas oven cooking at 350 degrees with poor ventilation produces as much carbon monoxide and nitrogen dioxide gas as is in the smoggy skies of Los Angeles.[3] Studies have also shown that a conventional gas range operating for a mere twenty minutes in a semi-closed kitchen can produce dangerous levels of these hazardous contaminants.

Carbon monoxide, an odorless gas, binds to red blood cells and thus deprives the body of oxygen. Exposures to low levels of carbon monoxide can cause headaches, blurred vision, nausea, dizziness, and respiratory problems.

Exposure to nitrogen oxides can cause light-headedness and burning sensations within the respiratory system. Recurring respiratory illnesses, such as colds and coughs, can be early signs of continual low-level exposure. In a study done at Harvard University Medical School of children ranging from ages six to nine, it was determined that those whose homes contained gas stoves suffered up to 15 percent more respiratory aliments than the children who lived in homes with electric stoves.

Microwave ovens also present problems. During my change to a nontoxic lifestyle, I postponed doing any research about microwaves, the working parent's best friend, until the very, very end. I correctly suspected that once I read about the risks associated with microwaves, I'd feel inclined to give mine up.

The first problem is that microwave ovens, and other appliances, generate large radio frequency levels. Since the human body operates by electrochemical activity, it is believed that changes in the earth's existing electromagnetic field can adversely affect our health. (I will discuss electromagnetic fields in more detail later in this chapter.)

Another concern with microwaves is radiation. There is a current debate over what is actually a safe level of radiation. If the microwave oven door is sealed tightly (and the oven is not leaking), then it probably is not giving off more radiation than is permitted by our government standards.

However, the standard of what is considered a safe level of radiation exposure is much lower in other countries. Researchers in the Soviet Union and other Eastern European nations have discovered that long-term exposures to low levels of microwave radiation specifically affects the central nervous system and can cause other conditions such as insomnia, decreased sexual potency, dizziness, and birth defects. In the Soviet Union and other Eastern European countries the acceptable radiation exposure levels are one-thousandth of the level considered acceptable in the United States.[4]

Asbestos in the Home

While many people may not have heard of many of the harmful chemicals present in our daily lives, most people *have* heard of asbestos, and most people know that it is something to avoid.

Asbestos is widely recognized as a serious health hazard. Since 1980, asbestos in building materials and products has been closely regulated. Individuals exposed to asbestos over a long period of time may experience coughing, shortness of breath, tightening of the chest, and sputum as early signs of disease. Continuous exposure may ultimately result in asbestosis, an irreversible scarring of the lungs that can be fatal, or mesothelioma, a cancer of the chest and abdominal linings.

Unfortunately, there are not any *immediate* effects of asbestos exposure, so individuals may not initially be aware that they are in any kind of danger. In fact, the diseases caused by asbestos accumulation may not appear for twenty years or more.

Asbestos can be found in almost any kind of building. In the home, materials such as plaster, ceiling tiles, insulation board, textured paints, and heating ducts may contain asbestos if they were installed prior to 1970. In addition, it is estimated that hazardous levels of asbestos still exist in approximately 35,000 schools.

People are exposed to asbestos when materials "shed" asbestos fibers as they become worn. Asbestos exposure can increase if the fibers are disturbed. Under no circumstance should asbestos be cleaned up by vacuuming. Vacuuming will just stir up and spread the fibers creating an even more hazardous situation. Cutting, sanding, or remodeling activities can also elevate concentrations of airborne asbestos. Since asbestos is more likely to be found in older homes, asbestos exposure should be an important consideration when doing any remodeling.

Radon in the Home

Lately, the media has focused much attention on a colorless, odorless gas called radon. Radioactive radon gas, which is produced in soil, can enter a home through cracks in the foundation or can diffuse directly into the home. Though not very frequently, radon can also be carried in water and then escape in the mist from washing machines, dishwashers, and showers. This type of entry occurs mostly in homes in northern New England.

When radon decays, it produces radon "daughters," bismuth, Polonium 218, Polonium 214, and Lead 210, airborne particles of which can get trapped in an individual's lungs. Once in the lungs, these particles decay even further, giving off alpha particles. Alpha radiation is the primary cause of tissue damage, which may then initiate lung cancer.

Presently, the EPA attributes between 5,000 and 20,000 lung cancer deaths a year to radon. As with asbestos, individuals are often not aware that they are being exposed to radon and there are no immediate known symptoms of radon exposure. Radon is not a problem affecting just a few, select homes. Studies by the EPA indicate that as many as eight million homes may have elevated levels of radon.

Electromagnetic Fields in the Home

Human beings are electromagnetic entities. Our living tissues generate electric currents, creating electric and magnetic fields. Since we are electromagnetic entities, we are influenced by electromagnetic fields. In fact, studies have shown that our body rhythms are tied to lunar and solar forces. However, when electromagnetic noise (which comes from artificial sources of electromagnetic radiation) interferes, our bodies have difficulty hearing the natural waves on which we are dependent. Many believe that exposures to strong electromagnetic fields can be dangerous to our health.

The total ambient electromagnetic field that you live in is the combination of those fields generated outside the house and those fields generated within the house. Outside the home, the levels of the ambient field will depend primarily on how close a home is to high voltage transmission lines and power transformers. Common sources contributing to the electromagnetic field inside a home are televisions, computers, microwaves, fluorescent lighting, and anything else that has a voltage transformer or an electrical motor.

It has been concluded by most studies that ambient fields greater than three milligauss (a gauss is a measurement of magnetic field strength) are linked to an increased risk of childhood cancer. Therefore, one milligauss for continuous exposures to 60-Hz fields is what is currently recommended since shielding a home from the ambient field is practically impossible. However, each of us can increase or decrease the field in and around our home by simply understanding what affects it.

For example, the television set distributes nonionizing electromagnetic radiation from the *entire* unit. It is a misconception that the electromagnetic field is only given off by the screen. Rather, since the box containing the circuitry is transparent to this radiation, the radiation is given off in all directions. In a study in which researchers placed lab rats twelve inches away from commercial television sets for four hours a day for thirty-five to fifty days, the electromagnetic radiation exposure which the rats received slowed growth, reduced the size of the male rats' testicles, and affected functions of the brain. In general, large-screen televisions produce stronger fields that will extend further out from the set.

In addition, fluorescent lighting produces a very different magnetic field than does an incandescent bulb. For example, a 10-watt fluorescent lamp produces a field at least twenty times greater than a 60-watt incandescent bulb.

A significant point to keep in mind when assessing exposure to electromagnetic fields is the amount of time one is exposed. This factor is especially important when one considers that many people are exposed to fluorescent lights all day long at their office or school.

Furthermore, size is not always important when determining how much of an ambient field an appliance produces. For example, a small bedside electric alarm clock can produce a field of five to ten milligauss at two feet away. If this clock is placed on a nightstand right next to the bed so that a person's head is within this range, the person will be getting considerable exposure all night long.

Hairdryers also generate very substantial fields. A 1200-watt model will produce fifty milligauss at six inches. However, since the average time spent using a hairdryer is minimal (with the exception of hairdressers who use them repeatedly throughout the day), the risk from hairdryers is not great. Fields as high as 200 to 400 milligauss have been measured one-half inch away from the cutting edge of a number of different electric razors. Each time the razor is used, the tissues right under the skin are exposed to this high magnetic field (remember: 60-Hz fields of only three milligauss have been linked to an increase risk of cancer). However, as with hair dryers, it has been argued that the overall risk from electric razors is reduced since the amount of time that one is exposed to this field is minimal.

This same argument, however, cannot be made about the field produced by electric blankets (fifty to one hundred milligauss) since exposure is usually not minimal as many individuals keep them on all night long. In addition, the concern over electric blankets is even greater since electric blankets are used very close to the body surface.

I cannot write a section on electromagnetic fields without mentioning that personal computers and video display terminals (VDTs) also present some concerns. The major difference between the hazards of a television set and those of a computer is that the computer operator is usually closer to the device. As I sit before my own computer and write this, I find myself scooting my chair backwards, noting that I am still not out of the range of concern (which is anything less than thirty inches).

Scientific studies done in Sweden and other European countries have researched the effects of computer radiation exposure on animals. For example, in 1986, Dr. Bernhard Tribukait and Dr. Eva Cekan of the Karolinska Institute, along with Dr. Lars-Erik Paulsson of the Swedish National Institute of Radiation Protection, reported that mice exposed to this type of radiation had five times the incidence of developmental malformations in their offspring than did the control mice. These results were confirmed by another study done at the Swedish University of Agricultural Science.

Additionally, doctors of Kaiser Permanente Health Group in Oakland, California, studied 1,583 pregnant women and concluded that female workers using computers for more than twenty hours per week had twice the miscarriage rate of female workers who did similar work but did not use computers. However, despite these studies and others, The International Radiation Protection Association still insists that "there are no health hazards associated with radiation or fields from computers or VDTs."

Personally, though, I am not going to bank on their advice. High on my list of things to do is to reduce my exposure to the electromagnetic field generating from my computer.

TOXINS IN COMMON PRODUCTS

Cleaning Products

Household cleaning products are among some of the most toxic substances we encounter daily. In one study conducted over a fifteen-year period, women who stayed home all day had a 54 percent higher death rate from cancer than women who had jobs away from the home. The study concluded that the increased death rate in the women was due to daily exposure to the hazardous chemicals found in household products including: ammonia, benzene, chlorine, formaldehyde, methylene chloride, naphthalene, toluene, trichloroethylene, and xylene. (The result of this study might suggest that women who complain that "housework is killing them" may not just be letting off steam.)

The average consumer may already recognize some of the more potent hazardous products, such as drain cleaners, but may overlook some other dangerous daily cleaning items. For example, ammonia carries warnings such as "POISON: May Cause Burns; Keep out of reach of children" or "CAUTION: Harmful if swallowed; Avoid inhalation of vapors; Use in a well-ventilated area." However, just about all popular commercial glass cleaners are merely a mixture of dye and *ammonia*, but I have yet to see a warning of any kind on a bottle of glass cleaner. Glass cleaners that come in aerosol containers are particularly dangerous since they distribute tiny droplets of ammonia into the air when sprayed that can thus be more easily inhaled.

The government acknowledges that cleaning products are hazardous and requires that they be regulated by the Consumer Product Safety Commission under the Federal Hazardous Substances Act. Yet, this regulation merely requires that warning labels, such as "corrosive," "combustible under pressure," "danger," "poison," "warning," and "caution," appear on products that can cause immediate injury or illness. However, most of these warning labels imply that the product is only harmful if it is swallowed. There is usually no mention of the adverse effects that result from inhaling toxic fumes or spilling the product onto one's skin.

Omitting this information seems rather absurd since clearly the mouth is not the only point of entry for dangerous chemicals. As fumes evaporate, they can be inhaled through the nose; many chemicals are easily absorbed by the skin. Just one square centimeter of skin contains 3,000,000 cells, 4 yards of nerves, 1 yard of blood vessels, 10 hairs, and 100 sweat glands. (My own new guideline is that if I would not want to drink something, why would I want to inhale or touch it?)

Cleaning products are not required by law to have full disclosure labels, which list EVERYTHING used in the product. Instead, manufacturers are only required to list their name and address, any active hazardous ingredients, a description of the product's danger, and instructions for storage or handling. But, as is the case with pesticides, manufacturers do not have to list any of their trade secrets on the label. Even the Consumer Product Safety Commission does not know what these secret ingredients are. Moreover, there is not a single government agency regulating approval of cleaning product formulations before they come onto the market.

Another point also came up repeatedly during the research for this book: although product labels provide medical advice on what to do if the contents are ingested, poison control centers warn consumers not to follow the advice. The poison centers encourage individuals to immediately phone their local poison center to get the correct information, since product labels often list incorrect antidotes.

Dishwashing and Laundry Detergents

According to the Center for Science in the Public Interest, dishwashing detergents are responsible for more household poisonings than any other household product.[5]

Chemicals that may be in your dishwashing detergent include naphtha, which is a central nervous system depressant; diethanolsamine, a possible liver poison; and chlor-o-phenylphenol, a metabolic stimulant that is considered very toxic. Another concern with detergents is the dyes used to color them. It should be noted that dishwashing detergents are not regulated by the FDA. In fact, according to consumer advocate Debra Dadd, there is basically no information that indicates that these dyes have ever been regulated for safety.

Laundry detergents may also contain hazardous chemicals. Perfumes, phosphorus, enzymes, ammonia, naphthalene, and phenol are just a few of the chemicals that can be found in some laundry detergents. Some detergents may also contain tetrapotassium pyrophosphate, a highly toxic chemical, and sodium aluninosilicate, which is sometimes used as a pesticide. Warning labels (e.g., "Harmful if swallowed" or "Keep out of reach of children") on laundry products could be considered further confirmation that many laundry detergents contain toxic chemicals.

Air Fresheners

Even prior to our change of lifestyle, I was suspicious of rooms reeking of air fresheners. Covering up odors with air fresheners does not change the fact that people in the room are probably still *inhaling* (though maybe no longer smelling) the source of the original odor. Simply, air fresheners do not "freshen" air; an opened window does that. Rather, air fresheners interfere with your ability to smell offensive odors either by releasing a nerve-deadening agent or by coating your nasal passages with an undetectable oil film.

Moreover, the chemicals used in a commercial deodorizer may actually be more harmful to smell than the odor that is being covered up. Commercial deodorizers may contain toxic chemicals such as methoxychlor, a chlorinated hydrocarbon pesticide that accumulates in fat cells and overstimulates the central nervous system. Likewise, P-Dichlorobenzene, naphthalene, and formaldehyde, all of which are central nervous system depressants, can also be found in some air fresheners.

Cosmetics

When considering the safety of cosmetics, it is first important to note that the seventeen-billion-dollar-a-year cosmetic industry is completely self-regulated by the CIR (Cosmetic Ingredient Review), a panel of independent toxicologists, dermatologists, and formulators. Since 1976, the CIR has reviewed 277 cosmetic ingredients and has concluded that p-hydroxyanisole (used in lipsticks) and chloroacetamide (used in moisturizers) are "unsafe under any conditions." However, more than 3,000 chemicals are used in cosmetic products. At a hearing in July 1989 on the safety of cosmetics, Representative Ron Wyden (D-OR) stated, "The FDA's existing authority to regulate cosmetics is no better than a toothless pit bull dog guarding a multimillion-dollar mansion." (Currently, the government is not even legally able to obtain information on specific formulations.)

At the hearing, numerous cosmetologists testified of symptoms such as headaches, loss of balance, memory loss, asthma, and irreparable nervous system and respiratory problems as a result of working with cosmetics. Because of these testimonies, a House subcommittee asked the National Institute of Occupational Safety and Health (NIOSH) to analyze 2,983 chemicals used in cosmetics.

The results were as follows: 884 of the ingredients were found to be toxic. Of these, 314 can cause biological mutation, 218 can cause reproductive complications, 778 can cause acute toxicity, 146 can cause tumors, and 376 can cause skin and eye irritations. The CIR has reviewed (or is intending to review) only 56 of these 884 ingredients.[6]

Since cosmetics are applied to the skin, toxic ingredients in these products can easily be absorbed. They can also be inhaled. The amount and type of damage a person receives from using cosmetics will vary depending on how much of the cosmetic is used, how often, and how well the person's detoxification system is working at the time. Here are just a few of the chemicals commonly found in cosmetic products:

- *Acetone*, a solvent which can affect the nervous and respiratory system, is used in nail polish remover.
- *Blue Dye No. 1*, used in aftershave and male cologne, body creams, blushes, and lipsticks, is a suspected human carcinogen.
- *Butylate Hydroxytoluene (BHT)* is found in lipsticks, baby oil, eyeliner pencils, and soaps. It is known to cause cancer in animals and is suspected to cause birth defects.
- *Formaldehyde*, commonly used in deodorants, antiseptic shampoos,

mouthwashes, toothpastes, nail polish, aftershave and perfume, is a carcinogen in animals and a suspected one in humans.
- *Triethanolamine (TEA)*, found in moisturizers, perfume, lotions, bubble baths, and hair gels, may combine to form nitrosodiethanolamine (NDELA), another potent animal carcinogen.
- *Lead Acetate* is found in hair dyes and is absorbed into the skin; it causes cancer in animals.
- *Methylene Chloride* can still be found in many cosmetic products, even though in 1985 the FDA recommended that it be removed from hairspray because it conclusively caused cancer in laboratory animals. (In fact, methylene chloride is so dangerous that two workers who used a product containing it to clean the Dirksen Federal Building in Chicago *died* after inhaling its vapors. The security guards who tried to rescue them had to be hospitalized and were still having headaches after being released.)

When reviewing the concerns associated with cosmetics, it should be noted that a favorite pastime of many young girls is to play "dress up," complete with Mommy's make-up and nail polish. Likewise, Mommy's cosmetics are sometimes used to add the final touches to a child's Halloween costume. A child will also inhale whatever cosmetic products his or her parents use. With these thoughts in mind, toxic cosmetics become a valid concern for children as well.

Talcum Powder

Even something as innocuous as talcum powder is suspect, because it may be contaminated with carcinogenic asbestos fibers. A study conducted by Boston's Brigham Woman's Hospital determined that women who used talcum powder on their genitals and on sanitary napkins were three times more likely to get ovarian cancer than women who did not use talcum powder.

Perfume

About 4,000 different chemicals are used to make perfume; as many as several hundred can be used in just one product. While the FDA is responsible for regulating perfume safety, it does not have the authority to require toxicity testing for it.

The primary organization in charge of doing perfume testing is the Research Institute of Fragrance Materials (RIFM). But, according to the National Academy of Sciences, RIFM does virtually no testing for neurotoxic effects, despite the fact that fragrance raw materials have been targeted as having a high priority for neurotoxic testing.

Symptoms triggered by perfume exposure range from headaches and sinus pain to anaphylactic shock and seizures. Some other commonly reported symptoms include: depression, irritability, memory lapses, inability to concentrate, and mood changes. Given these symptoms, one might wonder how productivity in the workplace (let alone children's academic performance in classrooms) might improve if people just stopped wearing perfume.

Soap

Even ordinary soap may contain hazardous chemicals. For example, several popular deodorant soaps contain triclosan, which is a relative of the pesticide 2,4-D and can cause liver damage.

The following chemicals may also be found in deodorant soaps: chloroxylenol (PCMX), clofucarban, dibromsalan (DBS), fluorosalan, hexachlorophene, phenol, tetrachlorosalicylanilide (TSCA), tribomsalan (TBS), and tricolcarban. The primary concern with these ingredients is that they can accumulate in the liver and other organs if deodorant soap is used daily.

As a person with multiple chemical sensitivities, I know from experience that soaps may contain potent chemicals. Not too long ago, my husband and I wanted to have some cabinets built for our laundry room. Since we were going to require specific nontoxic guidelines, it took several phone calls to find a carpenter who was willing to work with us.

I finally found someone who seemed most sincere. However, when the gentleman arrived at our home, I started having immediate reactions to HIM. More specifically, I believe I was reacting to the soap he used, since he looked and smelled like he had just showered. He was being so sympathetic about people with environmental illness while expressing a sincere willingness to make the cabinets with any specifications we wanted that I did not know how to tell him that, at that moment, HIS SOAP was causing severe reactions in me. To make matters worse, I kept trying to excuse myself by saying my husband would talk with him, but my husband, who was unaware that I was reacting to the gentleman, kept saying, "No, no, you said you wanted to be in charge of this project." I became convinced that I was reacting to his soap because on other days when he came over (and it did not appear like he had just gotten out of the shower) I had no reaction.

Dioxin Products

The word dioxin probably does not mean much to the average consumer. I certainly had never heard it mentioned in my other "toxic" life. Yet, the majority of consumers probably use products containing this chemical on a daily basis.

Dioxin, a very toxic substance which is a by-product of chlorinated compounds such as Agent Orange, is formed when chlorine is used to bleach brown wood pulp white. This bleached pulp is then converted into countless paper products such as diapers, sanitary napkins, paper plates, toilet paper, coffee filters, food packaging, and writing paper.

While dioxin's entire effect on humans has yet to be confirmed, immune system depression and impaired liver function have already been documented. The average person in the industrial world has measurable levels of dioxin in his or her fatty tissues as a result of dioxin exposures.

Besides the on-going human studies, there is conclusive evidence of the adverse effects of dioxin in laboratory animals. Studies have shown that even minute quantities of dioxin can cause miscarriage, liver disease, immune system depression, birth defects, and genetic damage in animals.

However, the paper industry (not surprisingly) states that the amount of dioxin in paper products is not high enough to pose any health risks to humans. Yet, despite the industry's reassurances that the levels of dioxin in such products as superabsorbent disposable diapers, paper towels, tea bags, tampons, juice cartons, TV dinner containers, and paper plates are too low to be of concern, there is evidence to the contrary.

For example, recent research shows that dioxin appears to migrate quite easily out of paper products. In fact, a 1988 Canadian study revealed that milk packaged in paper cartons (even those with plastic liners) contains consistently higher levels of dioxin than milk packaged in non-paper containers. Bleached coffee filters have also been shown to leach dioxin. In 1989, *Science News* stated that the two major sources of dioxin in paper products are milk cartons and coffee filters.

Presently, concern over dioxin has not yet motivated the average American consumer to advocate change. However, the situation is quite different in Sweden, where the paper industry and government have launched a successful consumer education program. It is now practically impossible for manufacturers to sell anything but unbleached, chlorine-free products in Sweden.

It is quite interesting to note what large manufacturers will do when their customers demand something. For example, all diapers marketed in

Sweden are now chlorine-free or have a very low chlorine content. When one major U.S. diaper manufacturer faced losing its share of the Swedish diaper market, the company began making chlorine-free diapers for export. Yet, the diapers they sell in the United States are still made from conventional bleached pulp.

TOXINS OUTSIDE THE HOME

Even if I had not repeatedly sprayed my home with pesticides, installed wall-to-wall toxic carpet and padding, or furnished the house with brandnew synthetic, formaldehyde-blessed furniture, there were still plenty of toxins in the area surrounding my home to cause numerous health problems.

One major source of toxins was the nursery across the street. I have no way of knowing how much its repeated spraying of pesticides contributed to my overall condition. I do know, however, that I spent many afternoons on our sunny deck and never gave a thought to what might be going on across the street. I also know that on the evening before my first emergency room visit a major fire occurred at this nursery in which sacks of banned, illegally-stored pesticides were burned.

Interestingly enough, the next afternoon I shared the emergency room with the eighteen firemen who had been fighting the nursery fire. Lying on a gurney, I could hear the emergency room staff discussing the firemen.

The doctors were clearly agitated when the chief, who knew that the firemen had been exposed to large amounts of illegal pesticides, requested that his men be examined. After much discussion, the ER staff finally decided that they would examine the three who were actually experiencing symptoms; the others were told to wait until Monday to see their own physicians.

Since I, too, was ultimately to be sent home without medical assistance, I now know that there were probably nineteen patients in the ER room that day suffering from pesticide exposure. Unfortunately, only three were given medical attention.

Even if the nursery had not existed, the road next to my home soon became another source of potential health problems. When we moved in, the street our house was on was very quiet. However, the city later opened up another street which, in turn, made our street a convenient shortcut. The traffic on our once peaceful street increased dramatically. In addition to the new noise pollution, we were also exposed to the hydrocarbons emitted from the numerous cars.

Then, just when I thought there could not be anything else toxic in and around my home, I started reading about high voltage wires. As I was reading about these big power lines, their description suddenly seemed quite familiar. So I found myself stopping right in the middle of the paragraph to look out of my window. I do not know why I was really surprised to see for the first time the high voltage wires behind my home. After all, I had already become convinced that my home was destined to with the "Most Toxic Home of the Year" award. In total, I think the only two sources of toxicity not associated with that home were asbestos and radon.

TOXINS IN THE NEIGHBORHOOD

Around Town

Regardless of how successful you may be at eliminating toxins from your home, you will undoubtedly still encounter them in various places around town. The shopping mall, a twentieth-century phenomenon, is a perfect example. With my chemical sensitivities, shopping malls are off-limits because of the toxic fumes, especially formaldehyde, outgassing from the new products. It did not surprise me to learn that shopping malls can have formaldehyde levels as high as 1.50 ppm (1.0 ppm is the level considered safe by the National Insititute of Occupational Safety and Health).

Another place where one might be exposed to a wide array of chemicals is the dentist office. While a trip to the dentist triggers apprehension in some individuals, for the chemically sensitive person, it is absolutely frightening.

Along the same vein, hospitals are equally frightening for the chemically sensitive patient. The chemicals outgassing from the cleaning and disinfectant materials used in hospitals cause reactions in many. Other chemicals that are commonly found in hospitals include formaldehyde, toluene, xylene, trichloroethylene, and hexane.

It is not just patients who may have adverse reactions to these chemicals. I know of several doctors and nurses who have had to leave their profession after becoming chemically sensitive to one or more of the chemicals used on the job.

Sick Buildings

"Sick building" is the term currently used to describe a structure whose occupants have health problems related to being in the building. A World Health Organization committee estimates that up to 30 percent of new and remodeled buildings may be sick buildings. This may not be surprising considering that OSHA admits that of the approximate 85,000 chemicals commonly found in the workplace only 600 to 700 have thus far been evaluated.

Sick buildings are a relatively new problem. They simply did not exist when buildings were made of wood, had lots of windows which were opened daily, had adequate ventilation, were furnished with natural materials, and were heated and cooled by natural sources. Today, however, windows are only decorations in energy-tight buildings. In addition, ventilation is poor, and plastic and synthetic building materials, which are often less expensive, have replaced natural ones.

One chemical which is known to contribute to creating a sick building is trichloroethylene. It can be found in carpet shampoo, floor polish, copy machines, and furniture glues. When trichloroethylene is inhaled, it enters the bloodstream and can then easily pass into lipid cell membranes. Common symptoms of trichloroethylene exposure are poor concentration and coordination, fatigue, numbness and tingling, headaches, and dizziness. (Not exactly optimal conditions to work under throughout the day.)

It should be noted that not all of the individuals working in a building need to be experiencing health problems in order to conclude that the building may be "sick." At the detox clinic, I met several people who became ill from working in a "sick building," like my friends Bill and Shelly, while others who worked in the same building appeared to be fine. However, just because the other workers were not manifesting symptoms at the same time does not necessarily mean that the building was not also having an ill-effect on them that might show up sometime in the future.

Unfortunately, long-term exposure to contaminants in a sick building may ultimately result in ill-health that persists even when the individual is away from the building. However, as a general guideline, individuals should become concerned if they start to notice a pattern of symptoms occurring when they enter a building and disappearing when they leave.

TOXINS IN THE SCHOOLS

While many sick buildings are offices, schools, which are often constructed with the same materials and energy-efficient guidelines as modern office buildings, can also become "sick." My husband and I were probably the only ones who were not thrilled when we watched a new elementary school being built down the road. Not only did school officials give no thought to what was going to be outgassing from the materials used, but the students actually began classes before the construction was completed.

My own daughter was supposed to begin kindergarten at this school six months after it had opened. After much discussion about the outgassing in the new school and some other considerations, we opted to send her elsewhere. We were aware that the school we chose to send her to was not toxic-free either, but it did have an administration that was willing to allow a group of parents to work together to make suggestions for reducing the amount of toxic chemicals in the classrooms.

Most parents have probably not thought about the harmful materials that might be present in their child's school. But I fear that if parents do not think about this, then no one else will either.

When I was a classroom teacher, my colleagues and I were committed to seeing that our students learned and developed to their maximum potential. Yet, I cannot recall one workshop, newsletter, or teacher evaluation that advised us on the role a *physical environment* could have on a child's health or learning.

I do remember watching many brand-new, windowless, carpeted portable classrooms come to the school, which were immediately filled with students. I also recall playground areas and classroom interiors being treated with pesticides. And, I have clear recollections of lots of fluorescent lights in every classroom and school building. In short, the school I remember would never qualify as an example of a nontoxic enviornment.

There are many sources of toxins in a school environment that can adversely affect one or more of the following: behavior, academic performance, and general health. One major source is the portable classroom used by many schools.

Portable classrooms are purchased or rented by many school districts because they are an easy solution to the problem of growing and changing student enrollments. However, portable classrooms are typically constructed from inexpensive (hazardous) materials and have little ventilation—two key factors that contribute to indoor air contamination.

Not long ago, a friend's son was placed in one of these portable classrooms. Soon afterward, the boy's academic performance went downhill dramatically. So drastic was the change that a conference between the mother and the principal was arranged. At this conference, the principal made a point of showing how the child's state testing scores had even dropped.

The mother was not that surprised. She had already begun to suspect that the materials used to construct the portable classroom were affecting her son. However, the idea that the *building* might be responsible for the child's change was completely foreign to the principal.

Yet blood tests confirmed that the son was having adverse reactions to the glues used to construct the portable classroom. After he was moved to a permanent classroom, his academic achievement improved to what it had originally been.

Other sources of toxins in the school environment that can affect health, behavior, and academic achievement include: cleaning materials, synthetic carpet, paints, pesticides, scents from the teacher (e.g., perfume, after-shave, hairspray), chemicals used in science lessons, mold, marking pens, glue, fresh newsprint, chalk, fresh asphalt, mimeograph or xeroxed paper, and fluorescent lighting. For example, a student's poor performance in math might be the result of a reaction to the vapors outgassing from fresh mimeograph paper on which his/her assignments are done. Perhaps a student is not trying to disrupt the class art project but, instead, is reacting to the marking pens, glues, and/or other materials used in the lesson. Likewise, maybe a student doesn't have eye strain but, instead, is affected by fluorescent lighting.(Fluorescent lights pulse on and off about sixty times per second. While we are not consciously aware of this flicker, evidence suggests that it causes eye strain, confusion, and can even impair one's judgement.)

The point here is to realize that many, many chemicals are present in classrooms and they may be affecting your child's academic performance as well as his or her health. In fact, Dr. Sherry Rogers, a prominent doctor specializing in environmental medicine, states that a common reason a child is placed in remedial class is not because the child has a learning problem, but because he or she has undetected sensitivities to chemicals and/or to food and molds (see chapter 6 for further information).

It seems to me that a profession dedicated to helping children learn would want to do everything possible to create the best possible learning environment. However, it may be that the personnel in your child's school are not even aware that they and their students may be exposed to dangerous chemicals and that these chemicals can affect a child's academic performance. Unless these problems are addressed, many children will continue to learn under less than optimal conditions. I assure you—even the best teacher and the most impressive textbooks cannot compete with persistent toxins.

SOLUTIONS AND ALTERNATIVES

Interestingly enough, it was not until we were in our new, nontoxic home that we realized how much the old house had affected the health of everyone in the family. Prior to the move, we had believed that the toxins in the home had only affected me, since I was the one who had become so ill.

However, some strange things happened after we moved into our nontoxic home.

In the old house, my husband's predictable morning sinus flare-ups were legendary. However, after residing in the new home just *one week*, his sinus condition disappeared.

Since our new home was only three miles away from our old one, we could not conclude that a different climate had prompted the change. Therefore, my husband's amazing recovery led us to ponder: Did my husband truly have a sinus problem—or was he, too, reacting to pesticides and formaldehyde?

His miraculously cured sinus condition was not the only notable change with our move. Almost simultaneously, everyone in the family suddenly required less sleep—about an hour and a half less than whatever each of us had been accustomed to. While my husband and I greatly appreciated that extra time each day, we were not quite prepared for our two-year-old to give up her naps. At first, not really realizing what was happening, we tried "forcing" her to take her afternoon nap. When it became obvious that she just was not tired during the day, we convinced ourselves that she would probably just go to bed earlier in the evening. No such luck. The girl just had more energy—and that was that.

REDUCING THE OUTGASSING OF TOXIC CHEMICALS

Everyone has heard of a cookout, but, in the future, the "bake-out" might become even more popular—especially if people continue to use materials containing toxic chemicals. In a bake-out, a building is completely closed up and the heat is turned on as high as possible. The building (or home) stays this way for as long as an entire weekend. The intense heat increases chemical outgassing by as much as 400 percent. This procedure usually reduces the overall chemical level in the house by as much as 25 percent. If you do this, be sure that the building is aired thoroughly before returning to it.

In addition to the bake-out, another way to reduce formaldehyde outgassing from cupboards and dressers is to apply a nontoxic sealant to the surface of any particle board. In our new home, it took my husband approximately two days to seal all the cupboards (see Appendix 2).

Entire rooms, such as attached garages, can be sealed off by using a vapor barrier. Auto exhaust and vapors from paints, pesticides, and fuels are just some of the common contaminants found in the garage that may be entering your home if your garage is attached to the rest of the home.

When we first moved into our nontoxic home, the attached garage presented us with a major dilemma. My husband, who had been very supportive of all the other changes in our lives, took his one and only stand when it came to the garage. He made it very clear that after three years of ingeniously parking three cars in a two-car garage, now that he had a three-car garage he was *not* going to park the cars on the street.

Luckily, we soon found out about vapor barriers, and our problem was solved. We simply tacked a vapor barrier all along the walls separating the garage from kitchen and sealed the seams with aluminum tape. (I admit it looks a little strange when the garage door is opened and one sees all this shimmering foil along the back wall, but we figured our neighbors already thought we were weird.)

For our vapor barrier we used Dennyfoil (Stock #242 or #245). Dennyfoil is virgin kraft paper with foil that is laminated with a sodium silicate adhesive on either side. It contains no petroleum products, fire retardants, pesticides, mold retardants or formaldehyde. Best of all, it seals off all vapors.

When separating a garage from the rest of the house, it is important to remember the shared ceilings/floors between the garage and the second story of a two-story home. In our old home, my girls' bedroom was right above the garage. In fact, a door from their room led to an attic over the garage. Vapors from everything stored in the garage easily drifted up into their room (toxic chemicals seem to show no respect for a closed door or a wall). Yet, if we had simply tacked a vapor barrier on the adjoining ceiling/floor, the vapors would not have been able to pass through.

Sealing and baking outgassing chemicals are not the only ways to reduce exposures. Those who like plants will be pleased to know that specific plants have been proven to significantly reduce indoor air pollutants. According to research at NASA's National Space Technology Laboratories, a small houseplant has been shown to remove up to 80 percent of some pollutants in a small, sealed chamber within a twenty-four-hour period. If a charcoal filter and small fan are added, the effectiveness of the plant greatly increases. In a tightly insulated 600-square-foot building outgassing formaldehyde and benzene, two eighteen-inch plants coupled with carbon filters and a fan reduced air pollutants to trace levels in forty-eight hours. The most effective plants for reducing air pollutants are spider plants, heart-leafed philodendrons, and elephant-ear philodendrons. (If adding indoor plants presents a problem to those with mold allergies, placing ground grapefruit seeds on top of the potting soil will help control the mold.)

Others may find it easier to eliminate odors and toxic chemicals by using a pale gray volcanic mineral called zeolite. Zeolite is completely nontoxic, has no smell of its own, and has multiple uses for improving air quality. Zeolite is effective in reducing contaminants because it has a negative molecular charge that attracts particles with a positive ion charge. The chemical structure of the mineral allows it to *adsorb* (meaning it holds gas or liquid molecules to a solid material). Examples of gases that zeolite can adsorb are formaldehyde, ammonia, hydrogen sulfide, carbon monoxide, and carbon dioxide. It can also adsorb smoke and bacterial odors.

Marketed under several trade names, such as Odor-Fresh and Non-Scents, zeolite comes in different-sized applicator bags and in shake-top cans.

A bag of zeolite in a closet can be effective in eliminating smoke, musty odors, and formaldehyde from clothing; in the bathroom it can be effective against toilet odors and mildew. It can also eliminate offensive odors from cat litter boxes and diaper pails. Likewise, zeolite can be used in any room or office to eliminate smoke, airborne odors, and some toxic gases.

I became very excited when I found out about zeolite. I thought it was great that there exists a natural, nontoxic solution to help reduce indoor air pollution. I also think that since zeolite is relatively inexpensive, more people may be willing to try this nontoxic alternative.

Last of all, OPENING WINDOWS whenever possible to provide natural ventilation will greatly improve indoor air quality. Toxic chemicals can be re-circulated for days in air conditioning and heating systems. In cold parts of the country where opening windows may not be feasible during the winter, an air-to-air heat exchange can be installed so that fresh air can come inside without your having to open a window (see Appendix 2).

Nontoxic (or Least Toxic) Furniture

After assimilating all the information regarding toxins in the home, we realized that furnishing our new home was going to present quite a challenge. Clearly, we were not going to be able to use any of our old synthetic, upholstered, pesticide-sprayed furniture. But, purchasing new synthetic items was no solution either.

After considering the alternatives, we decided to buy cushions and mattresses made from 100 percent organically-grown cotton and untreated wood frames. In one short word what that really meant was *futons*. There are probably more sizes and arrangements of futons in my new home than in some of the finest Japanese dwellings.

Futons made from organic cotton that has not been treated with fire retardants can be purchased from Dona Designs in Texas (see Appendix 2). The law requiring mattresses to be flameproof can be waived with a statement or prescription from a doctor. The clause which permits this waiver is paragraph 1632.1, "Standard for Flammability of Mattresses FS 4-72," of the Consumer Product Safety Commission's Flammable Fabrics Act Regulation. In addition to futons, Dona Designs also makes nontoxic mattresses and bedding, all made from organically-grown cotton.

It is important to note that many futon establishments advertise mattresses that are 100 percent cotton, but this does not necessarily mean that the mattresses are nontoxic. Aside from the fact that these mattresses have probably been treated with a flame retardant, cotton is sprayed heavily with pesticides when it is grown. For example, in Guatemala (where there are huge cotton plantations) a cotton crop can be sprayed as often as fifty times in a three-month growing cycle.

Nontoxic futon mattresses made out of untreated wool can also be purchased (see Appendix 2). Since wool is a natural flame retardant, it is not necessary to have a doctor's prescription to purchase these futons.

Purchasing bedding, mattresses, and cushions made from organically-grown cotton or untreated wool may be more expensive. But, I think that if there is one piece of furniture that really needs to be toxic-free, it is the bed. Personally, I cannot think of a better present for a child than a nontoxic bed—especially since that child is going to be sleeping there for nine to twelve hours every night for years. (Another advantage to our futon beds is that about once a month we put the futon mattresses outside in the sun to air out. Within a couple of hours, they literally "poof" up and look brand new!)

For those who remain skeptical, can I claim that our new couches look the same as a three-piece upholstered sectional or that my futon bed resembles a double-mattress synthetic king-size one? No. But are they comfortable? Yes!

However, if the "futon look" just does not suit your personal taste, there is another alternative—modifying your old furniture. You can reupholster your old furniture and replace foam rubber or synthetics with white cotton batting. Also, white barrier cloth can be used in place of upholstery fabric, and slipcovers can be made from untreated cotton, linen, or silk (which can be removed for washing). These materials can be purchased from The Janice Corporation, The Cotton Place, and Winter Silks (see Appendix 2).

As for tables, rattan, glass, and stainless steel are considered the least toxic. Since it is the finish that is the main source of toxicity in wood furniture, one solution is to purchase furniture made of unfinished wood and apply a nontoxic finish yourself. Beeswax (which can also be purchased from Dona Designs) is what we used on our unfinished oak kitchen table.

Alternate Flooring

The alternatives to wall-to-wall carpet are hardwood floors, tile, and linoleum. However, these too can be toxic if the proper materials are not used.

In our new home, we ripped out all the carpeting and vinyl flooring (much to the amazement of my new neighbors). When my husband pulled up the vinyl flooring in the bathroom, the vapors from the glue used to install the flooring were still so potent that he became nauseous, even though he has no chemical sensitivities.

Once down to the cement slab foundation, we put down a vapor barrier (the same kind we used to seal off the garage) to prevent both moisture and pesticide residues (practically all house foundations are sprayed with a pesticide before construction) from seeping into the home. We then laid our floor with wood that had never been treated with pesticides (from a special mill in Wisconsin, see address in Appendix 2). Instead of using glue, we opted to build a subfloor to which the wooden planks were then nailed. For the finish, we used a nontoxic product (Crystal Shield, see Appendix 2) that dried in approximately thirty minutes. To my amazement, I was immediately able to enter the home without having any adverse reaction. Our contractor was also amazed at the final results. He originally expressed concern over our choice of nontoxic materials, but, in the end, he liked the results so much that he wrote down how and where he could purchase these materials for future jobs.

When we were selecting the flooring, we did not choose hardwood floors for our entire house. Instead, we decided to use tile for the kitchen, family room, and bathrooms. Using the old-fashioned method, we simply laid the tile with Portland cement.

We also did not use any nontoxic linoleum in our house (see Baubiologie Hardware in Appendix 2), but others may find it useful. The product is called Natural Linoleum, comes in twenty-four different colors and has a life expectancy of forty years. It is an electrostatically neutral material so there is no problem with static build-up. The floor can be laid with AFM 3 in 1 Adhesive, a safe, nontoxic adhesive well-suited for use with Natural Linoleum (see AFM in Appendix 2).

While these nontoxic floorings are initially more expensive, I believe that in the long run they will prove cost effective. In our new home, I now never have to worry about cleaning my carpets. When my youngest drops her jelly sandwich face down on the tile, I merely smile. I know that a wet sponge will wipe it right up. Likewise, when my children and the neighborhood gang come running through with muddy feet, I can just sweep away the dirt after they leave. I honestly do not miss plush, wall-to-wall carpet.

However, to provide warmth and serve as sound barriers, 100 percent untreated cotton or wool throw rugs can be added. I have thus far only purchased two bathroom rugs (made from 100 percent untreated cotton from The Janice Corporation) because I have yet to find a cotton rug that has not been sprayed with pesticides or a wool rug that has not been mothproofed. In the interim, we have bought an exercise mat (also made out of 100 percent untreated cotton from The Janice Corporation) for our girls to do gymnastics on while our search for a nontoxic rug continues.

Realistically, I know that it is not likely that people will immediately replace their carpet with hardwood or tile floors. However, usually over a period of time, the need for new carpet arises. This might be the ideal time to start thinking "hardwood" and "tile" instead of "synthetic" and "chemically-treated."

Nontoxic Walls

Just about the only thing we did not re-do in our new home was the walls. Though they had not originally been painted with nontoxic paints, they had been painted almost three years ago. We concluded that daily ventilation and the use of an ozone machine (which can be rented or bought from Nigra Enterprises, see Appendix 2) would sufficiently alleviate the outgassing problem. Ozone, which is an oxygen molecule with an extra atom of oxygen attached to it, expedites the outgassing process by neutralizing pollutants. This plan seems to be effective because I can only still smell paint fumes if the house has been closed up for an extended period of time.

However, if you do decide to paint your home, there are nontoxic paints available. Unlike most commercial paints, nontoxic paints do not contain petrochemicals, mercury, formaldehyde, carcinogens, or toxic volatiles of any kind. When my parents recently painted their entire home with nontoxic paints, I was actually able to visit them *the day after* the house had been painted without experiencing any adverse reactions.

As for wallpaper, Elmer's paste or wheat paste can be used to apply the paper instead of traditional wallpaper paste. But there is still the problem of the pesticides and fungicides added to wallpaper itself. In our home, instead of hanging wallpaper, we covered the walls in our girls' bedroom with framed "masterpieces" of their own, original artwork. Actually, I think they get more compliments on this wall covering than they would on any wallpaper we could have selected.

Wardrobe Changes

Not surprisingly, clothing made from natural fibers, such as cotton, wool, and silk, is preferable to clothing made from synthetics. Unfortunately, natural fiber clothing may not always be the most practical choice—especially if one has young children.

Natural fiber clothing costs more than other clothing, and since children outgrow clothes so quickly, it may seem difficult to justify such an investment. Additionally, families in which both parents work might not have the time to iron natural fiber clothes. These factors are real considerations.

In our own household, wardrobe happens to be the one area in which we have not completely abandoned our old ways. If you were to go through my girls' closets, you would still find clothes made of synthetic materials—in fact, approximately 50 percent of their wardrobes are synthetic. Even given all I know about chemical outgassing, it is still difficult for me to justify spending the extra money on natural fiber clothing for my daughters since the clothes will most likely be outgrown, ripped, or stained within a matter of months.

But I also cannot deny what I know about synthetic clothing. Because our pre-schoolers are still changing sizes so often, we purchase both synthetic and natural fiber clothing. As our children get older, we will be more inclined to buy them only natural fiber clothing, which is what we already purchase for ourselves.

Some environmentalists and consumer advocates may believe that we have simply "rationalized" our way out of this dilemma. These same people would probably be even more surprised to learn that I recently purchased some "jellies" for my girls. (For those who are not hip in the under-twelve world, jellies are the new, *all plastic* shoes.) That I would purchase plastic shoes for my daughters may seem like a contradiction to some. However, to me, it is not. In fact, it is an example of a primary objective of this book.

Prior to learning about chemicals and toxins, I only considered size and color when I went shoe shopping for my girls. Not once do I recall thinking about chemicals. However, when I bought the jellies, I definitely considered that they are made of an unacceptable material. But when I weighed the amount of plastic in a small size eight shoe against all the other chemicals that we had removed from our children's lives, I decided to buy them anyway. Aware of the potential problems associated with the shoes, we, of course, did not let our girls keep them by their beds at night. In fact, for the first several weeks, the jellies were parked outside when not being worn.

So, yes, I bought shoes that were less than desirable from a chemical perspective. But the point is that I bought them *with knowledge*. I am no longer purchasing items with the blind belief that everything for sale is safe. I applied this thought process to a purchase that might seem insignificant to some (buying a pair of toddler shoes). Yet, parents know that it is the little, everyday choices that we are confronted with that ultimately make a difference.

Eliminating Pollutants While Cooking

Adequate ventilation is extremely important when using a gas range, since this helps remove combustion contaminants which arise during cooking such as nitrogen dioxide and carbon monoxide, and carcinogens such as benzol pyrone. Along with opening windows while cooking, installing a fan-operated range hood vented to the outside can help provide adequate ventilation. However, even with proper ventilation it is still very difficult to eliminate the small amounts of gas that escape each time a burner is lighted.

The Grand Microwave Elimination Plan

After I first read about the problems associated with microwave ovens (discussed earlier), we implemented stage one of the what turned out to be "the grand microwave elimination plan." In this first stage, we made a conscious effort to avoid standing directly in front of the microwave when it was operating.

In phase two of our plan, we moved the microwave from the kitchen to an adjacent, closed-off service room. We thought that if we couldn't see the microwave, then we would be less likely to use it. Also, we believed that placing the microwave in another room would reduce our exposure to its electromagnetic field. At that time, I did not yet understand that electromagnetic fields can travel through walls. I really thought our microwave was safe.

However, this plan went awry when we had our home tested for electromagnetic activity. The test results clearly illustrated the enormous impact our operating microwave oven had on the electromagnetic field of our house. When the testing instrument was placed directly in front of the microwave, the numbers indicating an increase in electromagnetic activity skyrocketed. In addition, even though the microwave was operating in another room, the test showed that its electromagnetic frequency still greatly impacted us when we stood in the kitchen. I think it was this demonstration that made me truly appreciate how powerful electromagnetic fields can be.

After this demonstration, we finally made the decision to get rid of the microwave for good. Surprisingly, despite all my past microwave dinners, instant boiling water, and baby-bottle warm-ups, my former microwave dependency is now only a blurred memory. I am pleased to report that after an initial "grieving period," I honestly no longer miss it. (Since then, I have become best buddies with the toaster oven, which I realize also contributes to the electromagnetic field—but to a lesser degree).

REDUCING OTHER TOXINS IN THE HOME

Reducing Asbestos Exposures

Since asbestos can be dangerous to remove, it is important to seek a trained individual to first help you determine whether or not asbestos is a problem in your home. To find such a person, call the EPA TSCA assistance line, (202) 554-1404, to find out if your state has a training or certification program for asbestos removal contractors and to receive information on the EPA's asbestos program. For questions related to businesses, call the Federal EPA Asbestos and Small Businessman Ombudsman's toll-free number, (800) 368-5888.

Reducing Radon Exposures

The most effective strategy for controlling radon exposures is to prevent the gas from entering a building or home. This can be done by increasing the structure's air pressure to levels slightly above those outside. Sealing foundation cracks, providing separate ventilating air to basements, and increasing ventilation rates are also helpful. In one case, when two basement windows of a home were opened and an exhaust fan was used, radon concentrations were reduced dramatically.

Testing your home for radon can be done for as little as fifteen to forty dollars (see Appendix 2 for information on radon testing). In Washington, Oregon, Idaho, and Montana, individuals may even be eligible for free radon testing. Individuals living in Pennsylvania may be eligible for state assistance for both testing and remedial action.

Reducing Electromagnetic Fields

Reducing exposures to electromagnetic fields includes determining the safe distances from any given field, using protective shields, and discontinuing use of electrical products that generate high fields. For example, computers should be placed at least thirty inches away from the user. Or, a computer shield can be purchased which protects users against the electrical field radiation. Baubiologie Hardware (address in Appendix 2) sells computer shields and a lightweight apron designed for persons who must work with electrical appliances on a continual basis (recommended especially for pregnant women). For offices, employers may want to purchase "The Safe Computer Monitor." It is somewhat expensive for home use, costing approximately $1,000 to $2,000. However, it is presently the only computer monitor that omits no magnetic, electric, or X-ray radiation. The Safe Computer Monitor works with most minicomputer and mainframe computers. (See Appendix 2 for where to purchase one.)

In the home, couches and chairs can be situated far enough away from television screens to be out of the range of the hazardous electromagnetic field. Heavy quilts can replace electric blankets, or beds can be warmed with electric blankets before one retires for the night. However, electric blankets must be *unplugged*, not just turned off, for the night since many blankets produce a field just by being plugged into the socket. In addition, battery operated alarm clocks can replace electric ones, manual razors can replace electric razors, and incandescent bulbs can replace fluorescent lights.

Dr. Edward Long of Humboldt, Kansas, describes how individuals can use a small battery operated AM radio to detect electric fields. (Although AM radios do not respond to magnetic fields, knowledge of an electric field can serve as a reasonable indicator of a magnetic field.) To detect the electric field given off by a television, first tune the radio to a spot on the dial where a station cannot be heard and turn the volume up all the way. Next, hold the radio about one foot away from the television when the set is turned on. You should hear noise coming from the radio. Next, slowly move the radio away from the television. There will be a distance at which the noise disappears. This is approximately the one milligauss level—the level considered safe. This method can be used to measure the electrical fields of other electronic items such as computers and stereos. However, it will not work with appliances, such as electric stoves and hair dryers, that only give off 60 Hz.

You can also purchase or rent an electromagnetic field meter. The "Safe Meter" from Safe Computing Company (address in Appendix 2) is an instrument which measures the magnetic components of 60 Hz and 1,500 Hz (VLF) fields. In some parts of the country, environmental consultants will come to your home or office and measure the electromagnetic fields. One such company is Safe Environments (address and phone number in Appendix 2), which presently has representatives in California and the New York metropolitan area.

PRODUCT SUBSTITUTIONS

Household Cleaning Alternatives

All toxic household cleaners can be replaced without having to sacrifice a clean house for a dirty, germ-infested one. Our grandparents did not have access to the vast array of cleaning products found in modern supermarkets, yet their homes were certainly clean—perhaps even cleaner than our homes today.

One of the benefits of using nontoxic cleaning alternatives is that they are much less expensive than toxic products. Presently, individuals can purchase nontoxic cleaning products from a variety of commercial companies (see Appendix 2), opt to make their own cleaners, or do both. For example, instead of traditional products, my nontoxic cleaning bucket generally consists of the following: baking soda (absorbs odors, deodorizes, and is a mild abrasive); distilled white vinegar (cuts grease, retards mold growth, and dissolves mineral accumulation); borax (disinfects, deodorizes, retards mold growth); and washing soda (cuts grease and cleans dirt). I also use a commercial non-chlorinated scouring powder (Bon Ammi) and Granny's Nontoxic All Purpose Cleaner (both companies listed in Appendix 2).

Nontoxic alternatives to household cleaners may initially seem strange, but after seeing how effective they can be, even the biggest skeptics have become convinced. Here are some creative alternatives to toxic cleaners:

DRAIN CLEANERS: Pour three tablespoons of washing soda down the drainpipe (followed by lots of water) several times a week. For unclogging, pour one handful of baking soda and one-half cup of white vinegar down the drainpipe. Cover drain tightly with a plunger for one minute. Repeat the process as many times as necessary.
DISINFECTANTS: Use a solution of one-half cup of borax to one gallon of water.
GLASS CLEANER: Mix two tablespoons of cornstarch and one-half cup of white vinegar in one gallon of warm water.

Metals can be polished with the following alternatives:
CHROME: Use apple cider vinegar on a soft cloth or rub the chrome with a lemon peel.
BRONZE, BRASS, COPPER, AND STEEL: Rub these metals with table salt dampened with lemon juice or vinegar.
SILVER: Rub with a paste made from baking soda and water or place in a pan and cover with sour buttermilk. Let the silver sit in the milk overnight and rinse with cold water in the morning.

Furniture, too, can be polished without using toxic chemicals. For example, oak furniture can be polished with a solution made from mixing one quart of beer that has been boiled with one tablespoon of sugar and two tablespoons of beeswax. Allow time for the mixture to cool and then wipe it on the wood with a dry chamois cloth. For mahogany furniture, mix equal parts of warm water and vinegar. After wiping this on the wood, polish with a dry chamois cloth.

These are just a few of the many alternatives available. Several organizations offer detailed information about nontoxic cleaning alternatives (see Appendix 2). The book *Clean and Green*, by Anne Berthold Bond (see Appendix 1), is an excellent, comprehensive reference guide of products and alternatives for nontoxic cleaning.

Air Freshener Alternatives

Besides using zeolite, some other ideas for freshening room air include: placing sachets of fragrant herbs or flowers around the home; leaving two teaspoons of vanilla or other flavoring extract in an uncovered container; setting out an open container of baking soda or a quarter of a cup of vinegar; and simmering lemon, grapefruit, or orange slices in an open pot.

Cosmetic Alternatives

If you have found some of the alternatives to toxic cleaners a bit strange, be forewarned that the following examples of effective substitutions for cosmetics may sound even more bizarre:

HAIR SPRAY: Chop one whole lemon and cover with hot water. After bringing it to a boil, keep boiling until half of the original quantity of water remains. Squeeze the lemon and liquid through a cheesecloth strainer. (It may be necessary to add water if it appears too thick.) This innovative lemon hair spray can then be stored in a pump valve dispenser and put in the refrigerator.

HAIR CONDITIONER: (for dry hair) - Blend together one-third of a peeled ripe avocado with one-third cup of mayonnaise. Massage mixture into scalp and hair. Rinse and shampoo.

TOOTHPASTE: Whip three-fourths cup of salt in a blender until it is pulverized. Then add three-fourths cup of baking soda and blend until the mixture is a very fine powder. For flavoring, some mint can be added.

As with cleaning products, these are just a few of the possible alternatives to using cosmetic products that contain secret (and more than likely untested) chemicals. If individuals are not interested in making their own cosmetics, several reputable companies, such as Aubrey Organics and Source Naturals, produce nontoxic cosmetic products that can usually be found in local health food stores.

Dioxin-Free Products

A few companies are now offering dioxin-free paper products (see Appendix 2). These products are usually found in health food stores. However, a major grocery store near my home presently carries dioxin-free paper towels and toilet paper. Purchasing products that have not been dioxin-bleached is not only less toxic for you and your family, but it sends a direct message to paper product manufacturers.

Paper products that are now routinely bleached would still adequately serve their purpose even if they were not bleached bright white. It seems reasonable to believe that an American market for low-bleach or no-bleach paper goods could be created if consumers began to demand and buy such products. Dioxin free products are both better for consumers and better for the environment. (Does it really matter what color toilet paper is?)

CURING SICK BUILDINGS

All of the suggestions that have been mentioned thus far for reducing the outgassing of chemicals in the home readily apply to curing sick buildings, including schools. Yet, before implementing changes, it is probably prudent to first discuss the actual problems of the building with whomever in management would ultimately authorize changes. People may be open to hearing about the possible problems with the environment of a building, but the issue of what it is going to cost to fix the problems will inevitably come up. However, it should be pointed out that after diagnosing a sick building, the implementation of remedial changes is imperative or health problems will undoubtedly continue. If the various changes recommended are considered "too costly" or "not top priority," those in the decision-making positions should be reminded that sick buildings, unlike human beings, have never been known to cure themselves.

It can be very helpful at this stage to have a list of suggested remedies *and* their projected costs. Likewise, management might be interested in learning the following facts presented in the EPA Report to Congress on Indoor Air and the subcommittee hearings on the Indoor Air Quality Act of 1989. This report concluded that indoor air pollution is one of the nation's most important environmental health problems. The report also concluded that improving indoor air quality is cost-effective since the annual national medical care costs resulting from indoor pollution may be as high as 1 to 1.2 billion dollars. The annual cost of productivity losses resulting from major illnesses due to indoor pollution was estimated at between 4.7 and 5.3 billion dollars.[8]

IN THE FUTURE

Changes *are* being made, and indoor pollution has become a major issue—and not just among environmental groups. For example, it is no longer uncommon to find articles on ventilation and toxic building materials in professional trade magazines.

In addition, some exceptional ideas are being implemented for improving the air quality in schools. For example, in Ontario, Canada, the Waterloo County Board of Education built a "clean" classroom, designed specifically for students and teachers with chemical sensitivities. In this innovative classroom, one cannot find plastic, carpet, synthetic curtains, odorous art supplies or chemically-treated paper. Additionally, the room is lighted by full spectrum lights, and no one smelling of perfume, tobacco or any other chemical is allowed to enter.

I also am encouraged that more people are becoming aware of the health problems associated with chemicals when I read notices like the one below, which appeared in an announcement for a National Women's Association conference: *Many women suffer from environmental illness, allergies, and asthma, and therefore we ask that all conference participants please refrain from smoking inside conference facilities. In addition, we ask that conference participants refrain from using artificially scented products, such as perfumes, hair sprays, and recently dry-cleaned clothes. These substances contain toxic chemicals that can cause severe allergic reactions.*

Although it is possible to get discouraged over the enormity of the indoor air contamination problem, keep in mind that, at least in the home, indoor pollution can be controlled. While I may not be able to directly improve what I breathe outside each day, I can control what I breathe inside my home. And that's where I am for a good part of my life.

It may be a long time before there are actual routine checks for indoor air contamination. Remember that the automobile emitted a lot of carbon monoxide for a long time before smog checks became required. It may take a while for the masses to become equally concerned about indoor pollution. But I am confident that it will happen. Luckily, each of us does not have to wait until then. We can begin making positive changes in our lives today since many, many nontoxic product alternatives already exist.

CHECKLIST FOR SUGGESTED CHANGES AND COMMITMENTS

☐ "Bake out" buildings/rooms which are outgassing numerous toxic materials.

☐ If the garage is connected to the home, seal it with a vapor barrier.

☐ Replace fluorescent lights with full incandescent lights.

☐ Begin to replace carpeted areas with hardwood, natural linoleum, or tile flooring.

☐ Hang spider plants or elephant philodendrons throughout the house.

☐ Avoid purchasing products made of pressed wood and/or particle board.

☐ Apply a nontoxic sealant to all particle board in the home to prevent the outgassing of formaldehyde.

☐ Use nontoxic paints.

☐ Purchase bedding made from 100 percent natural materials.

☐ Purchase a non-synthetic mattress.

☐ Purchase or reupholster furniture with natural materials.

☐ Purchase unfinished wood furniture and finish it with a nontoxic finish.

☐ Use nontoxic household cleaners.

☐ Use nontoxic polishes.

☐ Use nontoxic hygiene products.

☐ Use nontoxic cosmetics.

☐ Use dioxin-free paper products.

☐ Wash dishes with a nontoxic detergent.

☐ Launder clothing in a nontoxic detergent.

☐ Purchase clothing made from natural fibers (e.g., silk, wool, and cotton).

☐ Remove dry-cleaned garments from bag and hang in well-ventilated area for several days to a week before wearing.

☐ Purchase products that do *not* come in aerosol cans.

☐ Reduce and/or eliminate use of a microwave oven.

☐ Open windows when cooking.

☐ Organize a group to help inform school districts and businesses of the problems with toxins and the nontoxic solutions available.

☐ Organize a group to raise consumer awareness of dioxin in everyday products.

☐ Reduce exposure to electromagnetic fields by ensuring that family members are a "safe" distance away from the fields and by replacing electrical appliances with non-electric ones.

☐ If warranted, have your home tested for radon, asbestos, electromagnetic fields and/or formaldehyde.

Quiz 4—A Pretest on Food and Drinks

1. Peeling commercial fruit and vegetable skins _____.
    A) may remove some of the surface pesticide residues
    B) will remove all of the pesticide residues of the fruit
    C) will remove all of the surface pesticide residues but not any residues inside the fruit

2. Benomyl, a fungicide that has been classified as a possible human carcinogen (but which cannot be detected by the FDA's routine laboratory tests) is used on _____ food crops in the U.S.
    A) eight
    B) thirty-one
    C) forty-three

3. Out of the seventeen billion pounds of bananas imported to the U.S. between 1983 and 1985, the FDA tested a total of _____ samples.[1]
    A) 1,050
    B) 139
    C) 10

4. A legal source of "bottled water" is _____.
    A) tap water
    B) spring water
    C) well water
    D) all of the above

5. The word "natural" printed on a label legally means _____.
    A) nothing
    B) that only natural ingredients have been used in the product
    C) that only organic ingredients have been used in the product

6. _____ percent of all poultry, 90 percent of all pigs and veal calves, and 60 percent of all cattle (not including organic farms) are given antibiotics.
    A) Eighty
    B) Ninety-five
    C) One hundred

7. Approximately _____ cases of salmonella are believed to occur in the U.S. annually.
    A) 500
    B) 2 million
    C) 10 million

Answers to Food and Drinks Quiz

1. C   Peeling the skin will completely remove any surface residues; however, it will do nothing to eliminate residues found inside the fruit or vegetable.

2. C   This pesticide is of great concern because it is *systemic*, meaning that it gets inside the fruit (therefore making it impossible to remove the residue by washing, scrubbing, or peeling). Additionally, Benomyl causes birth defects and has been shown to decrease sperm count in test animals.

3. B   Between 1983 and 1985, the FDA analyzed 139 banana samples. During this time period, bananas were imported to the U.S. from fifty different countries. However, the FDA did not test any bananas from ten of the countries. Incomplete sampling of imported produce is of significant concern because imported produce frequently has twice the amount of pesticide residues than domestic produce. Additionally, imported produce may have been grown with pesticides that have been banned in this country.

4. D   Legally, "bottled water" is just that—water that comes in a bottle. There is no law requiring manufacturers to indicate the source of the water or if it has been treated. However, if manufacturers do choose to print where the water came from, for example, "Spring Water," then this information is supposed to be true. Bottled water with a label that simply reads "Drinking Water" might just be tap water treated with chlorine.

5. A   Manufacturers have quickly learned that labeling a product "natural" is an excellent marketing tool. However, the word "natural" on a product *legally* means nothing. While a product claiming to be 100 percent natural may or may not contain artificial colors, flavors, preservatives, or other synthetic additives, the product should not be considered *organic*. Organic foods are labeled accordingly.

6. C   In total, more than 1,000 drugs and another 1,000 chemicals are approved by the FDA for use in animal feed.

7. B   According to the U.S. Department of Agriculture, salmonella may be present in one out of every three chickens sold in the United States. Salmonella is most commonly found in raw meats, poultry, eggs, milk, fish, and products made from these foods. Symptoms (e.g., fever, headache, diarrhea, vomiting) usually appear within twenty-four hours; however, many people do not associate their symptoms with salmonella. Instead, they believe that they have just come down with the "flu."

CHAPTER FOUR

What We Really Eat and Drink

I returned home from the grocery store and placed the shopping bag on the counter. I reached into it and pulled out something for my two-year-old to see.

"Look, Kiley!" I called.

As soon as my daughter saw what I was holding, she began jumping up and down, exclaiming, "YIPPIE! YIPPIE!"

My new babysitter looked at both of us with disbelief. My two-year-old was ecstatic not over chocolate, ice cream, or donuts, but over carrot juice—freshly-squeezed, organic carrot juice.

My children were not born with organic, health-conscious taste buds. In fact, prior to my illness, it would have been fair to classify both my girls as popsicle junkies, whose primary diet consisted of hot dogs, snack crackers, and sugar-sweetened cereals. Our family's dietary changes did not happen overnight. It was a gradual process in which we slowly eliminated unhealthy foods and substituted them with healthy ones.

In fact, we were not even aware of our final transition until a neighborhood potluck supper in the park. As the dinner was spread out, we found ourselves looking with surprise at hot dogs, sodas, potato chips, and cupcakes. Suddenly, we realized that dinner for us was going to consist solely of our contribution (rice chips and tabouli salad).

Even more surprising was that my girls did not even want a bite of the cupcakes or a handful of the potato chips. Instead, they couldn't seem to get enough of the rice chips and tabouli.

Noting how content our girls were with this "strange food," one of the fathers started asking us about our eating habits. He wanted to know if it was difficult to eat only healthy foods.

My husband and I immediately responded, "No, not at all." But then I remembered more clearly the steps we had taken to reach this point. No, it hadn't always been so easy. Once upon a time—not that long ago—our family had also loved steaks, french fries, and sodas. And, as for sweets, my four-layered chocolate cakes, chewy brownies, and melt-in-your-mouth cookie creations had earned me the title "Dessert Queen." My husband was known to devour an entire strawberry cheesecake in one sitting, and at age two, my eldest became legendary one Christmas for polishing off an entire box of candy when no one was watching.

So, in looking back, I had to remember how and why we initially began to make some changes in our diet. In doing so, I recalled that sugar was the first of our old habits to go after reading about it in *Sugar Blues*, by William Duffy, and in several other books on Candida (which all stressed how sugar aggravates this chronic health condition). Next, it occurred to me while detoxing at the clinic how self-defeating it was to "sweat away pesticides" if I was still eating fruits and vegetables that had been sprayed with countless chemicals. So, we began to eat only organic produce. I was also becoming worried about all the growth stimulants, hormones, and antibiotics found in meat and poultry. I was especially concerned about the antibiotics since I knew they made Candida worse. These facts and concerns prompted us to begin eating only natural meat and poultry (animals which had not been given hormones or antibiotics).

Around this time, my acupuncturist's wife (also an acupuncturist) recommended that I eat a macrobiotic diet. To learn more about this diet, I read *The Macrobiotic Way* by Michio Kushi. The book includes numerous testimonies from people who had actually been cured of cancer after going on the diet. I was impressed. The book made a convincing case for how this diet could be instrumental to self-healing.

But the diet consisted of many strange foods that I had never heard of before, such as a variety of seaweeds: dulse, nori, wakame hijiki, and khombu. The book also describes a root called kuzu, a condiment referred to as gomashio, and plums (that did not resemble any plum I ever heard about) called ume plums. In short, the diet just seemed too bizarre to implement. Additionally, at that time, I was still too sick to do any cooking or shopping by myself, and I could hardly justify asking my poor parents (who were already running to special markets to buy us organic produce and natural meats and poultry) to now enroll in a macrobiotic cooking class. But, in looking back, I believe the macrobiotic seed was planted after reading that book.

Seven months later, I was feeling well enough to do the cooking and shopping. Moreover, I had progressed dramatically since my first day at the detox clinic, and I was hopeful that our new nontoxic home (we had moved in about a month before) would help me regain my health even more.

Yet, I still had countless medical problems, many of which were related to my digestive system. For example, when people would ask me what foods caused adverse reactions in me, I would tell them that it was easier for me to name the foods that I could eat, rather than those that I could not (since the latter was a much longer list).

Once again, I found myself thinking about a macrobiotic diet. This time, however, I read a book that did not make it appear so bizarre or difficult to implement. After reading *The Self-Healing Cookbook* by Kristina Turner, I became determined to give macrobiotics a try. I called up a macrobiotic restaurant and arranged a consultation with a macrobiotic counselor.

During the two hour consultation, my husband and I were given an informative, general overview of macrobiotics and suggestions for how to modify the diet to my own specific health condition. Best of all, at the end of the consultation, the counselor took us into the store section of the restaurant and showed us what each of the strange foods in the diet looked like. ("So, that's khombu!") We were encouraged to enroll in a macrobiotic cooking class, but I did not feel healthy enough to do this (the consultation alone was difficult for me since I still tired so easily back then). The counselor then referred us to a macrobiotic cook named Shelly, who agreed to come to our home to teach, demonstrate, and/or cook for us.

Not only did Shelly give me my first macrobiotic cooking lessons (several of which I had to view from the couch when I was not feeling well), but she also shopped for our pressure cooker, bamboo mats, salad press, and surachi—all items commonly used when preparing macrobiotic meals. In short, she got me started.

Almost immediately after beginning the macrobiotic diet, I started experiencing positive health results. The most significant change was in the amount of energy I had. This new level of energy was especially amazing considering how extremely weak and tired I had been for the past fourteen months.

As I write this, I have been on the macrobiotic diet for a little over a year. Interestingly, I find that I now have more energy than I ever had even prior to becoming ill. This really confuses the doctors because last year I was diagnosed has having hypothyroidism, a condition for which fatigue is usually the primary symptom. Yet, I am full of energy (and symptom-free) despite the fact that I have opted *not* to take any thyroid medication. In addition, if someone now asks me what foods cause adverse reactions in me, I can quickly respond since the list has decreased dramatically.

Without question, my personal dietary changes were initially motivated by my desire to get well. Even though I had made many changes in my lifestyle, it took me a while before I truly appreciated that food could also be a source of toxic contamination. But as I read and became more and more informed, I became more convinced of this. It was this conviction that prompted me to include the rest of my family in the diet changes I made.

Since I am sure most of my friends probably figure that I "force" my girls to eat this new way, it is my husband's new eating habits that really baffle them. They can understand why *I* might need to eat differently in light of my health condition. But, my husband is not sick and clearly does not have to depend on me for food. Moreover, there is nothing preventing him from indulging in treats at the office or snacking from the lunch room vending machines. My friends are intrigued to know why *he* chooses to eat in this strange manner.

His answer is very simple. Like my daughters and myself, he simply feels much, much better. He sleeps less and seldom catches a cold (and when he does, it passes within a day). And, he has come to truly enjoy the food.

Yet, as enthusiastic as I am about our new way of eating, I do not underestimate the great challenge it is to prompt others to even think about changing their eating habits. First of all, most people just do not want to know how their food might be harming them. After all, they enjoy their food, feel fine, and blindly believe that American food is unquestionably safe.

However, when planning our children's meals, it may not be fair to rely solely on blind faith. I believe that most parents would agree that ignorance is seldom a good guideline when making choices for children.

Even though I discussed pesticides in produce in chapter two, I include this more detailed chapter on food and drink because I now view both as yet another source of a variety of toxins which I hope parents will want to reduce from their children's (as well as their own) lives. I realize that most people do not think of food when they hear the word toxins. Likewise, I acknowledge that to think of food this way is both unsettling and scary. None of us likes to think that what we are eating and drinking might be having a poisonous effect upon our children or ourselves.

But the facts about the food we eat are so shocking and overwhelming that I believe I would have been remiss if I had excluded this chapter in a book about the toxins in our lives. In truth, I leave out a great many of the "gross" details and descriptions, since my objective is not to disgust anyone or make them ill. Instead, my objective is to inform. I believe it is imperative that parents have accurate, factual information about the food they are serving their families. I encourage and challenge you to objectively review all the facts presented here (without letting a craving for and/or a memory of a hot fudge sundae or a barbecued steak interfere) to determine if some of your family's eating habits may, indeed, need improving.

THE PROBLEMS

When looking at the typical American diet today, it is important to keep in mind that our grandparents (and most likely even our parents for the first half of their lives) never ate as we eat now. This is simply because food was different back then. Pesticides were not used on crops until after World War II; subsequently, *everyone* ate organic food. Likewise, poultry and livestock were not given antibiotics since they were not available until after World War II. Without "modernization," foods were not processed and tropical fruit stayed in the tropics. The average meal generally consisted of whatever was in season and grown locally.

In contrast, the overwhelming majority of food found in supermarkets today is processed and contains artificial flavorings, colors, and a long list of ingredients that most consumers have no idea how to pronounce, let alone whether or not they might have an adverse effect on their health.

The most pressing question about today's typical American diet is the long-term effects this diet is having on our health and that of our children. Clearly, no one is dropping dead after eating one burger from a fast food restaurant or one non-organic carrot. The problems associated with what we eat are not generally ones of immediate cause and effect. Unfortunately, this may make it easier for people to ignore the many problems associated with the typical American diet.

The food industry also makes it easy to believe that our diet is fine. This industry spends an incredible amount of time and energy on media campaigns designed to reassure consumers and make them feel good about what they are eating. The industry's campaigns are obviously effective since supermarkets typically have long lines of customers who feel confident that they are buying good, healthy food. That confidence, though, might begin to waiver if people were actually aware of some basic facts about the food industry.

THE FOOD INDUSTRY

As I was putting together the information for this chapter, I became concerned that many people might not believe some of the facts presented.

Therefore, I decided it was first important to provide some general background information about the gigantic food industry.

For example, impressive sources are always quoted to refute any questions over food safety. However, background information about the source is generally omitted. One very prestigious sounding source, The National Academy of Science Food Protection Committee, is actually independently financed by grants from commercial laboratories, chemical companies, and packaging companies. The Nutrition Foundation, Inc., another official-sounding organization, has board members from such companies as The American Sugar Company, Coca-cola, Beechnut, Campbell Soup, and General Mills.

The immense food industry has some other very influential members, such as the American Meat Institute, the National Livestock and Meat Board, the American Dairy Association, the National Dairy Council, the Cereal Institute, and the Sugar Research Foundation, Inc. All of these are national groups with ample amounts of money and lobbying power. Their official-sounding titles are *self-given*. However, carefully chosen words such as "council" and "institute" effectively portray these groups as unbiased.

For example, most people probably do not know (I certainly did not) that the concept of the Four Basic Food Groups taught to every elementary school child was, in fact, started as a promotion sponsored by the National Egg Board, the National Dairy Council, and the National Livestock and Meat Board. I do not remember ever being told that these boards and councils were the same people who would profit when these foods were bought.

Undeniably, the primary goal of the food industry has always been profit—not good nutrition for consumers. In fact, on the average, six cents of every dollar spent on processed food goes to buy advertising. Large companies, such as General Foods, spend approximately 340 million dollars a year on advertising. Moreover, the top fifty food firms control 90 percent of all advertising on television, of which almost half are commercials for cereals, candy, and gum. (Can you imagine an organic farmer competing for air time for a commercial about a non-processed, natural, organic peach?)

These mass advertising campaigns ultimately influence what we think about food. For example, I think it is interesting that so many Americans, who are typically not well-versed in nutrition, believe that milk is a rich source of calcium. Most would probably be surprised to realize that they know this fact simply because the dairy industry has told them so. A study done by the American Dairy Association indicates that an investment of 15 cents per farmer towards advertising produces a return of $1.68 in new revenues. Milk commercials are not public service announcements.

Unfortunately, the National Dairy Council has neglected to include in its media campaigns some other very relevant information about calcium. This is not really surprising, though, since the information would hardly increase milk sales. For example, the Council does not tell consumers about another mineral called phosphorus. Phosphorus can combine with calcium in the intestinal tract and prevent the absorption of calcium. Cow's milk is very high in phosphorus, while breast milk is very low in phosphorus. Although there are 1,200 mg. of calcium in a quart of cow's milk, compared to only 300 mg. in a quart of human milk, a breast-fed baby will receive more calcium by drinking breast milk because phosphorus inhibits the absorption of much of the calcium in cow's milk.

In addition, the National Dairy Council recommends a daily intake of 1,200 mg. of calcium to prevent osteoporosis, claiming that a calcium deficiency triggers this disease. However, there is evidence to contradict this. African Bantu women, who consume only 350 mg. of calcium a day and bear an average of nine children whom they breast-feed for two years each, hardly ever break a bone or even lose a tooth. When confronted with this information, the dairy industry has countered that genetics are the cause. However, studies show that when Bantu women come to live in the United States and consume the standard American diet, they have the same rate of osteoporosis as their American neighbors.

Regardless, the majority of Americans continue to drink lots of milk in order to prevent osteoporosis. However, many studies now indicate that not only does calcium not prevent osteoporosis, but that *high protein diets* (milk is high in protein) actually *cause* the disease. For example, Eskimos, who have diets very high in protein and who take in more than 2,000 mg. of calcium a day (from fish bones), have one of the highest rates of osteoporosis of any population.

The milk/calcium media campaign is just one of many media campaigns the powerful food industry sponsors. The information that the food industry provides (or chooses *not* to provide) usually goes unchallenged. Therefore, the average American naturally believes what he or she eats and drinks is safe.

One's family doctor often reinforces this belief in the safety of the food we eat, since he or she probably eats the same diet. However, it is important to note that during four years of medical school, the average physician receives approximately three hours of training in nutrition. It's not unlikely that many doctors are also influenced by industry media campaigns, just as many decades ago doctors even recommended that patients smoke as a way to deal with social anxieties.

WHAT'S REALLY IN BEEF, POULTRY, AND PORK

The meat and poultry industry is a very competitive business. Therefore, it should not be surprising to learn that hormones, drugs, and inexpensive feed are routinely used to help animals gain weight faster and/or to mask the signs of disease. Giving hormones and drugs to animals and feeding them inexpensive feed makes it possible for the animals to be bred and sold over a shorter period of time for the best profit possible. While these practices might be advantageous for the meat and poultry industry, they are not in the best interest of the consumer.

Growth Hormones

Hormones are naturally secreted by the glands of all animals (including humans). Only very minuscule amounts are needed to control an entire endocrine and reproductive system. However, additional growth hormones are routinely given to animals to introduce or delay fertility or to increase litter sizes. For example, when a sow is pregnant she will probably be injected with progesterone or steroids to increase the number of piglets in the litter.

While giving animals growth hormones may indeed increase the size of the litter and the size of the animals, there is a legitimate concern over how these growth hormones may affect the people who will eventually eat the meat or pork. According to Dr. Carmen Sanez, a physician in Puerto Rico, the effects can be quite shocking.

Dr. Sanez became worried when she started seeing a number of young children with precocious puberty. Some of the children she treated, some of whom were only four and five years old, had swollen or almost fully developed breasts. In fact, one five-year-old patient even had pubic hair, as well vaginal bleeding from a well-developed uterus.[2] Dr. Sanez suspected that these young children were, in fact, being contaminated by some kind of estrogen. However, she became confused when detailed patient histories ruled out the possibility that the children had used any medications or creams containing estrogen.

In February 1982, Dr. Sanez published her explanation for this outbreak of precocious puberty in the *Journal of the Puerto Rico Medical Association*. She stated that any neurological or other adrenal disorders had been ruled out as possible explanations for the children's symptoms. Instead, Dr. Sanez stated that she believed the premature puberty was the result of consuming local milk, poultry, and beef. Specifically, their symptoms were caused by the growth hormones administered to the animal and animal products that they had ingested. Dr. Sanez documented that when these children stopped consuming milk, poultry, and beef, most of their symptoms usually regressed.

While premature sexual development due to growth hormones in meat and poultry may be more prevalent in Puerto Rico than in the United States (partially due to the fact that the regulations regarding how many hormones can be given to livestock are not as enforced there), U.S. doctors are also seeing earlier puberty in American children. Likewise, it was stated in an English medical journal that hormone traces in meat were the reason English girls mature sexually at least three years earlier than in the past.

One particular hormone that is administered to livestock, DES, has caused great concern for years. Many people may already be familiar with DES. It has received extensive media coverage because of its proven link to a rare cervical cancer in the daughters of mothers who used the synthetic hormone as a fertility drug. DES is routinely given to livestock because it produces more fat and weight on the animals (and, thus, more profit). However, persons coming in contact with DES have noticed some very definite hazards associated with this hormone.

For example, ranchers have experienced sterility, atrophied testicles, and voice changes after inhaling DES dust.[3] The hormone has also been linked to breast cancer, fibroid tumors, and leukemia. In addition, researchers for the National Cancer Institute stated that only one molecule of DES in a quarter pound of beef liver may be enough to trigger cancer.

After a long political debate, DES was finally outlawed. Yet, just a few years after this ruling, the FDA discovered that approximately one-half million cattle were being illegally implanted with DES. In fact, according to John Robbins, author of *Diet for a New America*, DES can still be found in meat today. Furthermore, he claims that those ranchers not using DES have simply traded this hormone for one of the other sex hormones now on the market, such as Steer-oid, Ralgo, Compudose, and Synovexmany. Many of these hormones contain the same substances as DES. Robbins claims that sex hormones are used in practically every feedlot in the country.

Concern over these hormones is not consistent throughout the world. For example, in Europe, growth hormones are perceived to have such a negative health effect on the humans who will eventually consume the meat that the EEC (European Economic Community) in 1984 declared eleven major meat producers ineligible from exporting their products through the Common Market. The United States, however, still allows these companies to sell their meat in this country.

Drugs

Livestock consumes *more than half* of the twenty-five million pounds of antibiotics produced in this country annually. This is a 400 percent increase from twenty years ago. Penicillin and tetracycline are the two antibiotics most commonly given to poultry and livestock.

Repeatedly consuming meat from animals that have been given antibiotics may cause individuals to unknowingly become allergic to the antibiotics. *Annals of Allergy* reports the case of a fourteen-year-old girl who had anaphylactic seizures on four separate occasions after eating beef. When the girl was tested, it was discovered that she was not allergic to the beef itself but to streptomycin, an antibiotic. Her doctors concluded that the girl was reacting to the streptomycin residues in the meat.

Another concern is that toxic bacteria can build immunity to antibiotics. This resistance becomes encoded in the bacteria's extrachromosomal genetic material, which is then easily transferred from one bacteria to another. Therefore, when an animal ingests low levels of antibiotics, the number of resistant bacterial in its normal flora increases. Moreover, these antibiotic-resistant organisms are eventually transferred to the person who eats the meat or poultry. Once in the human, the resistant bacteria either colonizes in the human flora, or it passes the antibiotic-resistant genes to other bacteria living in the human body. The major concern about the transfer of resistant bacteria from animals to humans is that drugs which may be prescribed for the human sometime in the future may be completely ineffective when needed in life-threatening health situations.

One of the reasons antibiotics are given to animals is because the extremely crowded and poor conditions found on most factory farms today cause many animals to become sick. More than likely, the steak, ham or chicken on your plate did not first spend its life as a happy animal, roaming freely on the family farm. Instead, the animal probably spent its entire life in conditions not even remotely similar to the animal's natural habitat.

For example, the typical chicken today never sees sunlight or breathes fresh air. It spends its entire life in a twelve-inch-square cage with four other birds in a windowless shed completely controlled by computers. Not surprisingly, these kinds of conditions do not produce healthy chickens. Livestock are also bred in unhealthy conditions. Farmers and ranchers have come to rely heavily on drugs to ensure that their animals do not all die before slaughter time.

Pigs are also routinely given antibiotics and sulpha drugs to keep them alive. Modern enclosed pig pens are saturated heavily with ammonia to mask the stench caused by the horrendous conditions. This ammonia is then inhaled by the pigs day and night and gets into their lungs. It is estimated that over 80 percent of pigs have pneumonia at the time of slaughter.

The conditions in which cattle are shipped also encourage the use of antibiotics. The federal laws mandating under what conditions cattle could be shipped were written in 1906, before trucks were invented. Consequently, none of the guidelines pertain to trucks. Therefore, ranchers can avoid these federal restrictions by simply shipping their cattle via trucks.

Since no federal restrictions apply to trucks, conditions inside them can be very bad. Temperatures inside the trucks are either scorching hot or freezing (depending on the time of year), and there is virtually no ventilation. In fact, the conditions are so bad that cattlemen routinely expect some animals to die during shipping. They even calculate these deaths as part of their shipping expenses. Most of these deaths are caused by a form of pneumonia cattlemen refer to as "shipping fever." Since the Livestock Conservation Institute has stated that shipping fever ends up costing ranchers more money than any other animal disease, livestock producers are encouraged to rely heavily on an antibiotic called chloramphenicol to prevent it.

However, the FDA has grave concerns about chloramphenicol because it can, in a small but significant number of people, cause a fatal blood disorder called aplastic anemia. Only a minute quantity is needed to trigger this health condition in some people. According to Dr. Joseph A. Settepani, an FDA veterinarian who works in the area of human food safety, as little as thirty-two milligrams of chloramphenicol can kill a human being. This amount equals what would be found in one-quarter pound of meat with a residue count of eight parts per million. Some commercial beef treated with chloramphenicol has been found to have residue counts one hundred times that.

Animal Feed

In addition to antibiotics being added to animal diets, organochlorine pesticides are also found in feed grains. These pesticides can accumulate in very high levels in the fat of the animals. According to the U.S. General Accounting Office, 143 drugs and pesticides are likely to leave residues in raw meat. Forty-two of these are known to cause or are suspected to cause cancer, twenty can cause birth defects, and six can cause mutations.[4]

To understand why pesticides are so prevalent in animal products, it is necessary to look at how pesticides bioaccumulate up the food chain. Many people may be surprised to learn that one-half of the fish caught in the

world end up being fed to livestock. The problem with this is that fish absorb great quantities of toxic chemicals from the polluted waters in which
they swim (over 110 million pounds of DDT can be found in the oceans of
North America). The EPA estimates that fish can accumulate up to nine million times the level of PCBs found in the water in which they live.

In addition, fish have a long food chain. When one fish eats a number of
smaller fish, the bigger fish accumulates the total amount of toxins accumulated by the smaller fish. This process continues all the way up the food
chain. The cow, chicken, or pig that eats the feed made of fish then inherits
all the pesticides accumulated up the fish food chain. These toxic chemicals
are then passed on to the person who eventually eats the meat, poultry, or
pork.

Animals are also exposed to toxic chemicals that are absorbed through
their skin. For example, cattle, pigs, sheep, and other livestock are routinely
doused with the chemical toxaphene to kill the parasites that flourish as a
result of the unsanitary conditions in which the animals live. However, toxaphene, a chlorinated hydrocarbon, is a member of the same family as DDT.
Only a microscopic dose of this chemical is needed to trigger cancer and
birth defects in test animals. In other testing, it was determined that just a
few parts per trillion of toxaphene disrupted the reproductive function of
fish, while a few parts per billion turned the backbones of fish into chalk.
Yet, in spite of this, toxaphene is administered daily to animals.

The way in which toxins bioaccumulate up the food chain is of particular concern when we consider that we are at the top of the food chain. According to the EPA, food of animal origin is the major source of pesticide
residues in most people's diet. In fact, meat contains pesticide residues fourteen times higher than fruits and vegetables.[5]

However, pesticides and antibiotics are not the only things contaminating livestock and poultry. Animal feed may also contain sawdust laced with
ammonia, newspaper made with toxic inks, nitrofurans made from poisonous arsenic (which has been fed to poultry since 1950), and whatever else is
in the processed sewage, cement dust, cardboard scraps, tallow and grease
which are also routinely found in animal feed.

It took me a while to fully internalize that I when I eat meat, poultry, or
pork, I consume *everything* that the animal had consumed. After realizing
this, I chose to forgo even eating "natural" poultry, poultry which had not
been given growth hormones or antibiotics. Now, on those rare occasions
when I do purchase chicken, I buy only *organic* chicken—chicken that
wasn't given hormones or antibiotics *and* was fed only organic feed (See Ap-

pendix 2 for the addresses of mail order companies that sell organic meat, poultry, and pork.)

Inspection

In addition to the problems thus mentioned, other problems related to meat and poultry production may also be affecting our health. Consumers probably assume that unhealthy meat or chicken is not found in grocery stores, because it would not have passed government inspections. However, it should be noted that the United States Department of Agriculture (USDA) inspection process was established in 1906—long before modernization dramatically increased production.

Today, an inspector is typically allowed about three seconds to examine a carcass. The USDA only tests for toxic residues one out of every 250,000 animals slaughtered. And this test is only capable of detecting less than 10 percent of the toxic chemicals known to be present in meat. Even when hazardous levels are detected, the meat or poultry industry's reply is often that there is "no point in scaring the public." Such was its response in 1979 when PCB levels in the chickens of Ritwood Farms were so high that close to three million eggs and poultry products had to be destroyed. According to Lewis Regenstein, a well-established authority on pesticides, detection of these levels was actually unusual since most cases of PCB contamination go undetected and/or unreported.

Inspection guidelines may also surprise many consumers. The USDA relaxed its ruling regarding chicken inspection in 1970 because approximately 90 percent of all chickens are infected with the leukosis virus, a viral cancer peculiar to chickens. To help the industry compensate for this "economic hardship," chickens are allowed to go to market "if they do not look too repugnant." Tumors are to be "cut away," so the chicken can be sold as parts. To make diseased chicken look more appetizing, some feed contains artificial color to give the bird a "healthy-looking" skin.[6]

In addition to the large number of leukosis-infected chickens that pass inspection, according to an article in *Newsweek*, over one-third of the nation's chickens have salmonella. Salmonella poisoning is often mistaken for the flu since the symptoms are similar: cramping, diarrhea, and vomiting.

FOOD ADDITIVES

Additives are used in food either to aid in the processing or to improve the "quality" of the food. Common additives include nutrients, preservatives, artificial colors and flavors, anti-oxidants, emulsifiers, stabilizers, and thickeners. According to Letitia Brewster and Michael Jacobson, authors of *The Changing American Diet*, it is impossible to state exactly how many pounds of food additives Americans now ingest.

The food industry says food additives are completely harmless. However, government testing on food additives has never addressed the adverse effects additives can have on behavior, learning disabilities, or allergies. Likewise, the synergistic effect of additives is also not generally considered or tested.

However, the synergistic effect of food additives was very important in a study conducted at the Institute for Nutritional Studies. In this study, rats were given three combinations of three commonly used additives (sodium cyclamate, Citrus Red No. 2, and polyoxyethelene sorbitan monostearate). No effects were noted when the rats were fed only one of the three additives. However, when they were given a combination of Citrus Red No. 2 and sodium cyclamate, the rats stopped growing, developed diarrhea, and lost their hair. When they were given all three additives, the rats experienced rapid weight loss *and died within two weeks.*

Young children may be more susceptible to the adverse effects of food additives because their detoxification systems are not as effective as adults and because their brain and central nervous systems are still developing. Several studies appearing in medical journals have reported that the additive monosodium glutamate (MSG) can cause epileptic-like seizures in some children.

Artificial colors, another form of additives, are also of concern— especially since the use of artificial colors has increased elevenfold since 1940. Colors are commonly added to foods to make the food look more appealing. Over 90 percent of the colors used in foods are synthetic, usually coal-tar derivatives. Foods that are typically artificially colored include sweet potatoes, Irish potatoes, maraschino cherries, ice cream, candy, cake, frosting and fillings, butter, margarine, cheese, bologna, hot dogs, soft drinks, and oranges.

One artificial color that is commonly used is Citrus Red No. 2. Florida orange growers use Citrus Red No. 2 from October to December to literally *dye* green and spotty brown oranges bright orange. However, many leading food experts believe that Citrus Red No. 2 may be a possible carcinogen. In fact, as long ago as 1969, the FAO/WHO Expert Committee recommended that Citrus Red No. 2 no longer be used as a food coloring. At least eleven states (along with Canada) have banned the sale of artificially colored oranges. In states that do purchase oranges dyed with Citrus Red No. 2, grocers are required to post signs indicating that the oranges have been artificially colored. However, few stores comply with this regulation since enforcement of it is practically impossible.

The dying of oranges made a great impression on my nine-year-old nephew. In the past, my nephew had avoided making any positive statements about organic food for fear that it might somehow jeopardize his customary consumption of doughnuts and cookies. In fact, my nephew was quite vocal about his preference for *non-organic food*—until he found out about the oranges.

One evening, I slyly placed two oranges in front of him and said, "David, if you could choose between this orange (I pointed to one) that was picked off the tree when it was ripe or this orange (I pointed to the other one) that was picked off the tree when it was green and then *dyed* orange, which would you rather eat?"

Without hesitation, my nephew stated that he would want the one that hadn't been dyed.

"But, David," I said slowly, "that would mean you would prefer the *organic* orange. . . ."

Knowing he had been had, he looked up and smiled. But at the same time, his face portrayed a new awareness and concern regarding his past food preferences.

Other food colors have also been proven to be carcinogenic in animal studies. Additionally, artificial colors in food can trigger hyperactivity and behavior disturbances in some children.

According to Frances Moore Lappe, author of the best-seller *Diet for a Small Planet*, people should avoid eating food containing the following artificial colors: Blue No. 1, Blue No. 2, Green No. 3 (primarily found in beverages and candy), Red No. 3 (primarily found in cherries, candy and baked goods), No. 40 (primarily used in sodas, candy, sausage, and gelatin desserts), Yellow No. 5 (primarily used in candy, baked goods, and gelatin desserts), Orange B (used to color hot dogs), and Citrus Red No. 2 (used to color the skin of some Florida oranges).

According to Beatrice Trum Hunter, a renowned food additive expert and author, food dyes are particularly dangerous for young children since many of these dyes apparently pass easily through the blood-brain barrier. Noting the poor safety record of these dyes, she concludes that they should be banned. (Dyes have been used on a temporary, provisional basis for decades through extensions granted to the food, drug, and cosmetic industries.)

In addition to dyes, the following additives should also be avoided: brominated vegetable oil (BVO, found in soft drinks), butylated hydoxytoluene

(BHT, primarily found in cereals, chewing gum, and potato chips), sodium nitrite and sodium nitrate (primarily found in bacon, ham, hot dogs, lunch meats, and smoked fish), saccharin (used to sweeten diet products), butylated hydroxyanisole (BHA, found in cereals, chewing gum, and potato chips), MSG (used to enhance the flavor of soups, seafood, poultry, cheese, and sauces, as just a few examples) and aspartame (Nutrasweet, used to sweeten diet products).

Not all additives are harmful. The following additives are examples of some that are generally considered safe: agar, dextrin, lecithin, ascorbic acid, vanillin, hydrolyzed vegetable protein (HVP), and pectin.

In addition to colors, more than 1,500 flavors are also currently used to make processed food taste like natural food. These flavors are derived from petrochemicals. Firms such as International Flavors and Fragrances introduce more than 2,000 new flavors a year. These additives are usually just listed on the label as "artificial flavor" or "imitation flavor." As with artificial colors, artificial flavors can cause adverse reactions in individuals who are sensitive to petrochemical derivatives. Artificial flavors can also cause hyperactivity and behavioral problems in certain children.

Furthermore, "incidental" additives (additives that are never intended) can become part of our food from a variety of sources: pesticides, hormones, chlorine from bleaching processes, gas and solvent residues, polymers from plastic packaging, and lead cans. Lead soldered cans can increase the amount of lead that is leached into canned foods by 200 to 300 percent. The lead concentration can increase even more if the food is stored in the can after it is opened. This is especially true with acidic foods and fruits.

Sugar, another additive, is a major part of the American diet. Remember, too, that sugar has many aliases (e.g., corn sugar, dextrose), all of which can have the same negative effects upon the body as sugar.

At least with sugar, most people do acknowledge that it can cause tooth decay and can prompt hyperactivity (sugar highs) in children. Less well-known is the fact that sugar, as a simple carbohydrate, cannot be digested by the body without the help of other nutrients. To digest sugar the body needs to rely on nutrients from other foods, nutrients in the blood, and even nutrient reserves stored in the bones. On-going sugar consumption leads to an on-going depletion of nutrients.

The B vitamins, crucial to many body functions, are the nutrients most often depleted. The irony is that a deficiency of B vitamins *causes* sugar cravings.

Sugar also causes the pancreas to release insulin in an effort to combat the immediate rise of sugar in the bloodstream. However, if this quick stimulation occurs too frequently, the pancreas may begin to overreact (produce too much insulin) and/or will eventually lose the ability to release the correct amount of insulin necessary to metabolize carbohydrates.

Sugar intake can also make a person more susceptible to illness since sugar inhibits the ability of the white blood cells to fight bacteria. This fact did not surprise me because I can remember my husband always getting sick right before, on, or after Christmas. It is difficult to ignore that the month of December is usually full of an endless supply of sugar-filled treats. (We have now celebrated two Christmas holidays without sugar, and, interestingly, both holidays passed without so much as a sniffle from my husband.)

Most people generally accept that sugar can be harmful. The problem seems to be in getting people to acknowledge that sugar does not just appear in cookies and cakes. Many parents conscientiously monitor the amount of sweets their children eat. But, at the same time, parents often overlook the amount of sugar found in other processed foods. Sugar can even be found in condiments, such as ketchup, salt, and salad dressings!

I remember my surprise when I first began reading labels in an effort to consciously avoid all foods with sugar. A quick trip to the grocery store turned into an afternoon marathon as can after can, package after package, did not make it into my shopping cart because the food contained sugar. It was even the second ingredient listed on the label of my favorite brand of canned tomatoes!

After learning about sugar and the powerful food industry, I was intrigued to see the following headline in a national magazine: "The Latest Word on Sugar: It Won't Hurt You." The article actually stated that sugar "triggers no major disease, makes few if any people fat, and doesn't make kids climb walls." (The article did, however, concede that sugar contributes to tooth decay, but "no more than other foods.") The article quoted the doctor who had headed the FDA's "Special Sugar Task Force," which had concluded that any previous indictments against sugar were in error.

A few years ago, I probably would have read this article and then eagerly reached for my morning Danish roll with a clean conscience. However, as I read the article now (and continued to eat my organic whole oats cereal), I could not help but notice that the article appeared in November—just a few weeks before Thanksgiving and a few more weeks before Christmas. To me, it seemed unlikely that such earthshaking news being released at this holiday (sugar-filled) time of year was a coincidence.

While I must confess that I had no real knowledge or proof, I started speculating that this task force might be a clever marketing strategy to increase sales of sugar-filled holiday treats. Given what I had come to learn about the food industry, it did not seem unreasonable to question who may have originally initiated the creation of a "Special Sugar Task Force" and why. My doubts were further reinforced when I recalled the variety of sources I had read that greatly contradicted the task force's findings. Pondering these thoughts as I happily continued eating my organic whole oats cereal, I was pleased to note that I was now applying some critical thinking to printed information, rather than just automatically believing whatever I read.

Many individuals have decided to substitute artificial sweeteners for sugar. However, artificial sweeteners may cause even greater harm than sugar. Most Americans are currently consuming more aspartame than is considered safe. When the FDA approved aspartame for use in soft drinks, the agency did not know that aspartame would be used in thousands of food items as well.

Aspartame is of concern because it affects the brain by either increasing or decreasing the levels of various neurotransmitters. According to Dr. John Olney, a professor at Washington University, a young child who daily drinks several sodas sweetened with aspartame may have already consumed enough of this additive to possibly induce a brain lesion. However, the damage to the brain might not show up until years later, when any connection to aspartame would be unlikely. Even more frightening is what happens when aspartame and MSG are combined. Dr. Olney found that each additive enhanced the other, increasing considerably the total level of neuro-excitation.

In addition to aspartame, other substitutes for sugar include fructose, honey, and maple syrup. However, there are concerns with these alternatives, too. Despite the fact that fructose is often found in products in health-food stores, it is essentially no healthier than sugar. While it is somewhat easier to metabolize, it is still high in corn syrup, which is 55 percent sugar. While honey is generally not contaminated with insecticides (the exposed bees don't make it back to the hive), it is primarily composed of fructose and glucose. And, although maple syrup comes from the sap of trees not grown with fertilizers or pesticides, formaldehyde pellets are often legally inserted into maple trees to increase the flow of sap.[7] There is no law that requires manufacturers to notify consumers of this practice on product labels.

MILK

If you want to truly stun someone, just tell them that you have eliminated all dairy products from your children's diet. When I tell people that our family no longer consumes dairy products, it's as if I've said that I tear

American flags for dust rags. It seems it is just simply un-American to question—let alone negate—the merits of milk. (I have already discussed how effective the dairy industry has been in convincing us of the benefits of milk.)

However, since my family and I decided to give up dairy products, five of my friends have also decided to give them up. Like us, each of them has experienced a notable positive impact on their health. Specifically, they claim to have better digestion, fewer sinus problems, and healthier skin. These changes may not seem so surprising, however, when we look at some of the problems regarding milk.

One of the concerns is that milk can cause symptoms in people who are lactose intolerant (unable to digest lactose, the sugar found in milk). Among certain ethnic populations, the number of lactose intolerant individuals is staggering. For example, 90 percent of all Filipinos and Thais do not have the ability to properly digest lactose, while 85 percent of all Japanese, 78 percent of all Ashkenazi Jews, and 70 percent of all African-Americans are lactose intolerant.

However, persons who are lactose intolerant often do not know it, and, therefore, may not realize that drinking milk is the cause of their abdominal problems. In a study of children with recurrent abdominal pain (the "belly-ache" is a common complaint among children), one-third of the children turned out to be lactose intolerant. When milk and all milk products were removed from their diets, their symptoms disappeared.[8]

Lactose intolerant individuals may not be the only ones affected by milk and other dairy products. Milk can contain bacteria from the fecal matter that often contaminates a cow's udder and teats. Not all bacteria is removed with pasteurization. Government regulation requires that the level of bacteria in milk be kept to a minimum, but it does not require that milk be sterile. In addition, milk and dairy products contain five and a half times more pesticide residues than produce (unless the cows have only been given organic feed).[9]

Recent studies have also shown that much of our milk supply contains traces of potent, harmful drugs. Before drugs became an integral part of diary farms, a typical lactating cow could produce about 2,000 pounds of milk a year. With drugs, dairy cows can now produce an average of 14,000 pounds a year. Moreover, cows from some herds produce an average of 25,000 pounds a year, while some cows actually produce an incredible 50,000 pounds a year.

However, the demands placed on cows to produce huge, inordinate quantities of milk make the cows more prone to disease. Diseased cows are routinely treated with antibiotics and sulfa drugs, since dairy farmers do not want to have their cows out of production. The concern is that if humans are repeatedly exposed to antibiotics in dairy products, they may build up an intolerance to antibiotics. If this happens, then antibiotics given to that person in the future in an emergency situation may be ineffective.

In all, it seems fair to conclude that milk in the United States today is very different from what out parents or grandparents drank. To argue the merits of milk without acknowledging these facts seems remiss—especially considering the amount of dairy products ingested by the average American.

WATER

Most Americans avoid drinking tap water when abroad, but many people believe that the water in this country is perfectly safe. Unfortunately, this assumption is not always correct. Our water supply today contains numerous pollutants that municipal water treatment facilities were never designed to deal with when they were built in the early 1900s.

Water is still disinfected by adding chlorine to municipal water systems. However, some cities have had to significantly increase the amount of chlorine added to their water because of the spread of nitrates and phosphates from agricultural runoff. For example, over the past thirty years Chicago has increased the amount of chlorine in its water by more than 75 percent.

Although it is added to disinfect water, chlorine itself may make the water hazardous to drink. The EPA's Health Effects Research Lab (HERL) has found that two cancer-causing agents form in water when chlorine interacts with humus (the organic material resulting from the decay of plants). The first agent, called MX, has shown up in every chlorinated drinking water tested for it. MX is believed to induce genetic mutations. DCA, the other agent, can alter cholesterol metabolism and cause cancer. According to many scientists, MX and DCA are the most hazardous substances found in American drinking water today.

The amount of chlorine in the water supply may or may not be obvious to the people using or consuming it. However, now that I have multiple chemical sensitivities, I can easily detect chlorine in water. (I've been likened to police dogs that can sniff out drugs.)

I recently had the opportunity to use this unique new talent when I went to pick my daughter up from her friend's house. When I arrived, my daughter said that she needed to use the bathroom before we left. As soon as we entered the bathroom, I was immediately overwhelmed by the smell of chlorine and instantly began to have a reaction to it.

Leaving the bathroom as quickly as I could, I told the mother that I must have been reacting to some kind of chlorine cleaner that she had stored in the bathroom. But when she said that she did not have any cleaners stored there (and even went to double check), she began to wonder what the source of the chlorine was that I was smelling. I agreed to go back in the bathroom briefly to see if I could determine where I thought the chlorine was coming from. It turns out that I was reacting to the water in her TOILET.

The mother then turned on the water at her kitchen sink and asked if I would smell it too. While the smell of the running water was not as overpowering as the toilet water in the bathroom, there was no doubt that it also smelled like chlorine. When my daughter and I left, the mother had a very worried expression on her face and said that she intended to do something about her water.

Chlorine is not the only substance that can contaminate water. Water can also be contaminated with bacteria and viruses (usually from animal fecal matter), inorganic chemicals (e.g., arsenic, asbestos, cadmium, lead, and nitrate), and organic chemicals (e.g., pesticides, herbicides, vinyl chloride, benzene). All of these come from a variety of sources such as industrial wastes, landfills, and agricultural runoff. The degree to which water is contaminated can depend largely upon whether or not the water supply is close to city dumps, toxic waste dumps, agricultural fields, or industrial factories.

Currently, the EPA only monitors the levels of eight inorganic chemicals and ten organic chemicals found in water. However, the agency has identified more than seven hundred pollutants that can be detected in water. Of these, at least twenty-two are known to be carcinogenic.[10] The potential hazards of some of the other pollutants are unknown since they have not undergone testing.

Water can also become contaminated from the pipes through which it is transported. Water is often referred to as a universal solvent because it picks up a little of everything that passes by—such as calcium, copper, lead, and asbestos which may be in the pipes. Therefore, a report describing the condition of water at the source may not accurately reflect the condition of the water coming out of the faucets in your home.

Lead Contamination in Water

While many people may already be aware of the dangers of lead contamination in water, the EPA estimates that 25 percent of an average child's lead intake still comes from drinking water. (For infants, it is as high as 40 to 60 percent.) Municipal systems do test for lead, but the testing is done at the *source* of the water supply. However, over 90 percent of all homes and apartments in the United States have lead in their plumbing which can contaminate the water. Additionally, recent scientific studies show lead to be a health hazard at even *lower levels* than previously thought.

A recent study demonstrated how irreversible damage from lead can be. Dr. Herbert Needleman first became concerned about undetected juvenile lead poisoning back in 1959, when he was the chief resident at Philadelphia's Children's Hospital. In the 1970s, with the cooperation of school officials, teachers, and parents, he collected baby teeth from 2,300 elementary school children. He also gathered reports from teachers and parents on the behavior and learning development of these children. Sadly, Needleman found that those children with high levels of lead in their teeth scored poorly on IQ tests. These children also had poor verbal skills and short attention spans.

In 1990, Needleman reported the results of a follow-up study done on 132 of the children from the original group who had high lead concentrations. The study showed that these children had high school drop out rates that were seven times greater than those of students with low levels of lead concentration. In addition, these students had high absentee rates, reading problems, motor difficulties, attention deficits, and other neurological problems.[11]

Lead, in any amount, accumulates in certain body tissues and does not appear to be spontaneously eliminated over time. Lead is also known to migrate from a pregnant woman to her fetus, possibly initiating lead poisoning in the child before it is born.

Case studies of children exposed to lead have linked even low levels of exposure to shorter stature, impaired hearing, and impaired formation and function of blood cells. Many children will have no symptoms of lead poisoning, while others may have only non-specific symptoms (e.g., headaches, muscle aches and cramps, rashes) which can mimic other conditions. Severe lead poisoning can lead to coma, kidney damage, or serious brain damage. Lead poisoning has become such a widespread problem that the Center for Disease Control recommends that all children between the ages of six months and six years be tested for lead poisoning.

Lead in School Drinking Water

One memory from my teaching days is the purified water cooler sitting in the corner of the teachers lounge. In contrast, I also remember hundreds of children lining up each recess to drink from one of the school's water fountains. When I think back to those days, a question comes to mind: If the water in the fountains was not considered good enough for the adult staff, why, then, was it considered good enough for the growing children?

The more I started thinking about this, the more I thought it important that school districts be aware of the contents of the water consumed daily by hundreds of small children. I was greatly pleased to discover that the EPA had recently addressed the problem of lead in school drinking water.

The EPA is primarily concerned about lead in school drinking water for two reasons. First, even minute doses of lead can permanently impair a child's mental and physical development. Second, schools, by nature of their schedules, have an on-again, off-again water use pattern that can result in elevated lead concentrations. When schools are closed during weekends and vacations and over the summer, drinking water remains stagnant in the interior plumbing. This extended contact with the lead solder or pipes can result in elevated lead concentrations in the water.

According to the EPA, lead gets into water by one of two ways, either by being present at the source, or through the corrosion of lead parts in the distribution/ plumbing system. Typically, the latter is responsible for the lead in school drinking water. Experts say the corrosion of lead solder in plumbing systems is the primary cause of lead contamination in drinking water today.

Widespread lead contamination in school drinking water is likely if one or more of the following is true: A) the plumbing system is less than five years old and lead solder was used in the construction, B) the water is corrosive, C) lead is in the sediment in the plumbing and screens, D) lead pipes are used, and E) the service connector is made of lead.

Localized contamination, in which only some of the drinking water in a school is contaminated, is likely if: A) the water is non-corrosive, B) some locations in the plumbing system have lead pipes, C) recent repairs/and or plumbing additions used materials containing lead (e.g., solder, brass), D) numerous solder joints have been installed, and E) water coolers have tanks lined with lead or other construction materials made of lead.

After reviewing the above information, parents might for the first time find themselves wondering about the specifics of the plumbing system at their children's school—especially considering the fact that the water in both old and new schools can have high levels of lead. At this point, I feel compelled to mention a recurring thought I have had while writing this section. Unquestionably, while researching this book, the limitations of our government's ability to assess hazards and protect citizens has become quite apparent to me. So, upon discovering that both a law and an agency (the EPA) are urgently advocating remedial actions to reduce lead in school drinking water, I can only conclude that the problem is of *great significance*.

SOLUTIONS AND ALTERNATIVES

After reading the facts thus presented, you may feel overwhelmed and somewhat confused. And you may be wondering just what (if anything) is left to eat or drink. The good news is—there is PLENTY.

DEFINING A HEALTHY DIET

I fear that some readers may still think that their families *are* eating good, well-balanced meals. After all, their family is not drinking sodas, eating canned spaghetti, munching on doughnuts, or surviving only on TV dinners. Rather, in the course of a day, a typical family may have eaten the following: French toast with maple syrup, sausage, and orange juice for breakfast; grilled cheese sandwich, potato chips, and a piece of fruit for lunch; and steak, salad, and corn on the cob for dinner.

But, upon further examination we discover that the French toast was made with bread that contained white flour, preservatives, additives, and sugar. The "maple syrup" was, in fact, only 2 percent maple syrup and 98 percent chemicals and sugar. The orange juice came from oranges which had been dyed.

The grilled cheese sandwich for lunch was made with the same white bread as the French toast. The cheese contained pesticide residues. The fruit also contained pesticide residues and had been waxed.

The steak for dinner contained growth hormones and antibiotics, the corn on the cob was frozen and processed, and the salad was made with vegetables sprayed with multiple pesticides (more than 100 different chemicals are permitted on tomatoes, 75 on cucumbers, 60 on lettuce, and 50 on carrots).[12]

When evaluating how nutritional food is, you cannot just look at food names. The amount of pesticides, additives, preservatives, and artificial colors and flavors also need to be considered. For example, orange juice made from organically-grown oranges is a great source of Vitamin C and a nutritious drink. However, non-organic orange juice containing numerous additives and pesticide residues is not so nutritious.

Another factor to consider when evaluating your family's diet is whether or not it contains many foods that are either very alkaline or very acidic. It is an established fact that if the body becomes too alkaline or too acidic, coma or death can result. To prevent this, our bodies have a buffering system that keeps our pH factor (our alkaline and acid factor) balanced near 7.43. For example, after you eat salty meats, your body will try to balance itself by craving something sweet. (In fact, all cravings are the result of the body at-tempting to balance itself.)

But maintaining a pH balance of 7.43 is stressful on the bodies of people who eat the standard American diet. This is primarily because the American diet includes many foods that are either too alkaline or too acidic, such as red meat, dairy products, alcohol, and sugar. When you continually eat al-kaline or acidic foods, your body must expound a tremendous amount of energy to keep itself balanced, energy which otherwise could be utilized to promote health. Long-term problems that can occur as a result of the body having to perform a constant balancing act include lessened adaptability to the environment, premature aging, and the onset of chronic health condi-tions.

Therefore, it is desirable to eat foods which are neither too alkaline nor too acidic. By doing so, the body does not have to exert energy to keep itself balanced and can use this energy instead for self-healing. Examples of bal-anced foods are *whole* foods such as grains, vegetables, and legumes. When I first began eating a balanced diet, I could not understand why eating "whole foods" is so important. (What was wrong with my *rolled* oats?) I learned that whole foods are not processed and, therefore, contain all of their original nutrients and vitamins. From a nutritional perspective, whole oats are better than rolled oats, whole barley is better than pearled barley, and so forth.

In general a menu of balanced foods might look something like this (as-suming everything is organic): whole oats cereal, raisin bread, and carrot juice for breakfast; vegetable soup, rice, and an almond butter sandwich for lunch; and a salad, whole barley with steamed vegetables, lentil beans, and a fruit-sweetened cookie for dinner.

I know what you're probably thinking—that the menu above includes the kind of food you have always associated with those "health-nuts." After all, that's probably what I would have thought just a few years ago. How-ever, after eating this way and seeing the incredible health changes in my family and myself, I am now a firm believer in the impact diet can have on a person.

My beliefs are further reinforced after reviewing studies comparing the strength and endurance of individuals who eat high protein/fat diets with those of individuals who eat vegetable and grain diets. In a Danish study in 1968, a group of men were fed three different diets, after which their endur-ance on a stationary bike was measured. The men first ate a vegetable and meat diet. The average pedaling time on the bike before the men started ex-periencing muscle failure was 114 minutes. Next, the same men ate a diet high in meat, milk and eggs. After being on this diet for an equal period of time, the men were only able to average 57 minutes on the bike before experiencing muscle failure. Finally, the men were fed a strictly vegetarian diet, consisting of grains, vegetables, and fruits. The results after eating this diet were dramatic: the men were able to average 167 *minutes* on the stationary bike before experiencing muscle failure.

Medal winning performances by international athletes also confirm that high protein diets are not necessary for strength and endurance. Dave Scott, who follows a primarily vegetarian diet, has won Hawaii's legendary Ironman Triathalon six times. Other vegetarian athletes include Bill Pickering, who set the world's record for swimming the English Channel; Stan Price, who holds the world's record for bench press in his weight class; and Ridgely Abele, who has won eight national karate championships.

Since we changed our eating habits, my husband has improved his own performance as a part-time triathlete. In fact, my husband has a triathlete friend, almost ten years his junior, who has become somewhat flabbergasted over how fast "the old man" is racing these days. He is so amazed at my husband's new capabilities, he recently asked if he could come over for dinner to find out more about my family's diet.

There are numerous books that fully explain why and how to implement a whole foods diet. *The Self-Healing Cookbook*, by Kristina Turner (see Appendix 1), is an excellent, beginning resource. (Keep in mind that the balanced eating described in this and other books does not even remotely resemble the "balanced" diet presented by the food industry.)

Beginning Guidelines

I believe it is impossible to expect a child to eat healthy foods while Mom and Dad munch away on potato chips and ice cream. Even the smallest children are not going to accept "it isn't good for you, but it's all right for me." If parents insist on indulging in unhealthy treats, these goodies should be consumed when the kids are not around.

When introducing new foods, we discovered that it was easier to do so if the food being introduced was not presented with the rest of the meal. Somehow, placing the new food on the plate with the rest of the meal only seemed to encourage our daughters to devise creative ways of making the new food conveniently disappear via an amazing amount of squishing, mashing, and hiding.

Instead, we always introduced the new food first, on a separate plate or bowl. My children were never required to eat it. If they did not want it, that was fine. However, if they were interested in eating the rest of the meal, then they needed to first eat the new food. We also made sure that portions, initially, were very small.

Each of my children went through one meal in which they refused to eat the new food and chose to forgo the entire meal. On these occasions, we did not get angry or insist that they eat the new food. We simply reminded our children that before they were served anything else, they needed to eat the new food. Whether it was eaten before this meal or the next was up to them.

But even my own mother thought I was horrible when I served my daughter her leftover broccoli (on the same plate from dinner) the next morning for breakfast. However, I was willing to continue presenting those few stalks of broccoli for breakfast, lunch, and dinner all week if necessary—but I did not have to. Kids are smart. When my daughter saw that we were really serious, she ate the broccoli (which took approximately sixty seconds). Now, one year later, she loves it.

MAKING THE SWITCH

I would not recommend a "cold turkey" approach when changing your family's diet. You will be more successful if you implement slow, gradual changes with the long-term goal of ultimately eating only healthy food.

Be realistic and make the first change in just one area of your diet. Consider these starting points:

- avoid fast food restaurants
- buy meat and poultry that does not contain antibiotics or growth hormones
- do not buy foods that contain additives or preservatives
- do not buy food packaged in lead-soldered cans.

Another (although very ambitious) change would be to avoid eating all foods containing refined sugar.

As you implement these changes, you can slowly introduce some new nutritious foods at meals, gradually phasing out less healthy foods. Organic whole grains (e.g., rice, rye, barley) can complement just about any meal, and preparation consists of merely boiling water and measuring the grain. Listed below are some healthier foods which can be substituted for other commonly eaten foods:

- rice crackers in place of crackers containing sugar
- tofu dogs in place of hot dogs
- popsicles made from organic juices in place of commercial popsicles
- rice chips with no additives/preservatives in place of potato chips
- soy cheese in place of dairy cheese
- soy milk, rice milk and almond milk in place of dairy milk
- soy "bologna" in place of cold cuts
- organic fruit-sweetened cereals in place of commercial cereals sweet-ened with sugar
- organic fruit-sweetened cookies in place of commercial cookies sweet-ened with sugar
- carrot/raisin mana breads in place of sweet rolls
- soy and/or rice bean ice cream in place of dairy ice cream
- organic, no preservatives/no additives bread in place of commercial bread
- organic fruits and vegetables in place of non-organic produce
- purified water (*not* in a plastic container since the plastic leaches into the water) in place of just about any other drink
- moist, hand-harvested sea salt in place of refined salt

These substitutions can compliment a diet of whole foods; however, keep in mind that grains, vegetables, and legumes are recommended as the primary foods to be eaten. Also keep in mind that *organic* whole foods contain higher levels of such minerals as calcium, magnesium, potassium, sodium, boron, manganese, iron, and copper than grains, vegetables, and legumes that have been sprayed with multiple pesticides. For example, one study showed that organic snap beans contain 227 parts per million dry matter of iron, while inorganic snap beans have only 10 parts per million. Similar differences were noted for the other minerals found in the beans and for other vegetables as well.

Those who are still worried about eliminating dairy products (because of an ingrained fear of calcium deficiency) should be pleased to learn that there are many other good sources of calcium, such as broccoli, kale, collard greens, soy products, kidney beans, almonds (my kids now love almond milk), and sea vegetables. One cup of milk contains 288 milligrams of calcium (though we now know that this is not equivalent to how much will ultimately be absorbed). However, there are 136 milligrams of calcium in one cup of broccoli, 290 milligrams in one cup of collard greens, and 626.4 *milligrams* in one cup of hijiki (a seaweed used in many dishes).

For those people who are already shaking their heads, thinking that they will never be able to get their families to eat collard greens and hijiki, they may be in for a surprise. After eating a diet of whole foods, my family's tastes have changed dramatically. In fact, my family now fights over the collards and has actually come to enjoy hijiki in grains and vegetables.

For those who fear that they will never eat anything sweet again, be assured that naturally sweetened foods taste very sweet if not in competition with sugar desserts. Barely malt and rice syrup can also be used to sweeten food, because, unlike sugar, fructose, and honey, the body can digest these without depleting essential nutrients.

Most of the foods I have listed can easily be found in most local health food stores. They will probably cost somewhat more than their counterparts—if one looks only at dollars and cents. However, if one evaluates what one is truly getting for the money, then I believe the substitutions are actually the better buy.

The Excuses

By now, you might have come up with a list of reasons why this new diet—despite the facts and information presented—will just not work for your family.

"The health food stores are too far away."

"My husband will absolutely never change what he eats."

"You don't know *my* kids—they are stubborn and strong-willed when it comes to what they eat."

"I've eaten my old way for (X amount of years) with no problems."

"I can't afford health food prices."

If you are looking for excuses to continue eating as before, there are plenty. However, considering that so many Americans seem to end up with cancer, heart problems, arthritis, diabetes and more, you might want to reconsider. According to the World Health Organization, the United States rates only twelfth in a ranking of the health of nations in the world. Clearly, there is room for general improvement in the American diet.

As far as strong-willed children go, I must point out that if Webster had known my youngest, he probably would have written "See Kiley Green" next to the definition of stubborn. But being committed to helping your child change his or her eating habits is like anything else. If parents believe it is important, they will go to any lengths necessary.

Parents who claim they cannot get their child to eat certain foods surely face the same strong-willed child in other situations—like bedtime or crossing the street. Yet, somehow parents seem to find a way to enforce rules in these situations, because they know that allowing a child to stay up until midnight or to run into the street is not in the child's best interest. If the same perspective and energies are applied to guiding a child to eat properly, parents may be amazed at the results.

ENJOYING A HEALTHY DIET

Three New Food Categories

As old foods were phased out of my family's diet, we had a chance to acquire some new tastes. I felt it was important to provide ample heath food "treats" (e.g., organic, fruit-sweetened cookies or popsicles made from organic juices) so that even initially the "healthy foods" would not only be associated with the "yucky foods." When my children devoured their dinosaur-shaped organic cookies, we would take the opportunity to point out that we were now eating food that both tasted good and was good for us. We never denied that sugar cookies and cakes tasted good; we merely emphasized that it was possible to eat foods that were both tasty and healthy.

I ended up dividing all foods and drinks into three categories. These categories seemed to make a lot of sense to even my preschool-aged children. There were the "No-thank-you" foods (candy, ice cream, etc.) which not only did not nourish us, but were unhealthy; the neutral foods (rice chips, soy bologna, etc.) which were neither bad nor exceptional in their nutritional value; and the POWER FOODS (organic grains, legumes, vegetables) which made us strong—inside and out.

Calling the highly nutritional food "POWER FOOD" seems to be very appealing to my girls. Now, as they plow through their lentils, they identify them not as "yucky food," but as their "power food." One day, shortly after categorizing foods in this manner, my girls ran up 109 steps from the beach to the street. Barely out of breath, my eldest turned to me and exclaimed, "Wow! That food really does give me power!"

Even my daughters have noticed that since we changed our diet, they have stayed very healthy. In fact, for the first nine months after changing our eating habits, my children did not have one runny nose —let alone a cold, the flu, bronchitis, ear infections, or any of the other illnesses that plagued their friends (and used to plague us). This is in spite of the fact that my children were still surrounded by dozens of children every day, and, thus, exposed to countless germs (since a typical preschooler's idea of hygiene is to wipe his or her nose with a finger and then hug a friend).

Peer Pressure

When we first changed our eating habits, we thought that our children might experience some peer pressure and negative reactions from their friends. However, quite the opposite has happened. For example, our next door neighbor, who our preschool girls worship because she is almost six, loves our different food. When we invited her to lunch at our house, one would have thought we had asked her to dine at the most elite restaurant in town.

On the morning of the day that she was to eat with us, her mother told me that they had passed a fast food restaurant, and her daughter had asked if they could eat there. When her mother reminded her that this was the day she would be lunching with us, her daughter quickly said, "Oh, I forgot. Well, Callan's food is better anyway!"

Another neighbor of ours, a ten-year-old girl, readily admits that it is no coincidence that she often shows up at our house around dinnertime. She is quite open about the fact that she, too, loves to taste whatever we may be cooking. In fact, she has even on occasion invited some of her friends over so that they can watch her proudly identify the names of the sea vegetables. At least once a week, this wonderful ten-year-old-sent-from-heaven tells my girls how lucky they are to have this food and how she wishes her Mom would prepare it for her.

I don't really have an explanation for these girls' great enthusiasm. They both eat the typical American diet in their homes—complete with refined sugar, white flour, and preservatives. Other friends of my children who have come over have also happily indulged in our food. Two of my children's friends labeled "picky eaters" by their parents have cleaned their plates at our house.

I can only conclude two things—first, the food tastes good (fresh organic vegetables do not even compare with the frozen, contaminated variety) and, second, our own enthusiastic attitude about our new food just rubs off on our guests. For example, when a young friend sees my two children jumping up and down because they are going to get some pumpkin seeds or carrot chips, they naturally join in the excitement.

However, I have noticed that if the visiting child's parent is along, then the child is not as enthusiastic about the "new food." I believe this is because parents tend to transfer a lot of their own food preferences to their children.

Some parents may even subconsciously convey messages that reinforce "unhealthy" food. For example, I have yet to hear a parent say, "If you eat all your ice cream, I'll let you have some carrots!" But, the reverse is heard all the time. A subtle message is reinforced that carrots are yucky and ice cream is good.

That is why I think it helps to use a term like "power food" to explain the order in which food should be eaten. You can tell your children that "power foods" are eaten first because they are the most important. This approach then subtly changes the idea that it is necessary to suffer through undesirable food in order to get to the "good stuff." Instead, the reverse is expressed—the "good stuff" is eaten first.

We are not so naive as to believe that our children will never be subjected to peer pressure to change their eating habits. However, it will be just that—peer pressure—not a craving or a desire for a food that my children simply do not eat anymore. I believe that we will deal with those situations as we will deal with all the other cases of peer pressure that arise when raising children.

However, we believe that partly due to our new eating habits, our children may actually be less susceptible to peer pressure as they grow up. Since our children are presently so comfortable with being "different" and have such an incredible understanding of cause and effect and the human body, they may, in fact, be less vulnerable to peer pressure to use drugs, alcohol, or indulge in any of the other parent nightmares.

Respecting Each Individual's Choice

When offered food that our family no longer eats, we have taught our daughters to merely say, "No, thank you." We have been very careful to stress to our children that it is not our place to judge anyone by what they eat. It is an individual decision.

When we see someone indulging in something we have come to believe is "taboo," we point out that either the person does not yet know what we have come to learn (I repeatedly remind the girls of our "darkness" period when I fed them popsicles and hot dogs) or the person does know but chooses not to make dietary changes.

We use my own father to illustrate the latter case. Despite three rounds of cancer and shopping in all the health food stores for me when I was ill, he still eats bacon, sugar-frosted flakes, and other unhealthy foods. However, we stress to our children that we still respect his choice of food, just as he respects ours. Our primary point is that regardless of what other family members or friends choose to eat, our love for each other never changes.

For All Those Special Occasions. . . .

I would be untruthful if I did not say that it is a continual challenge to eat differently than the rest of America. The holidays, especially, test imagination and commitment. Below are my suggestions for dealing with some special occasions.

HALLOWEEN—Our children still dress-up, go trick-or-treating, and fill their bags with tons of artificially colored and flavored, refined-sugar candy. But when they return home, they dump their treats onto the kitchen table and begin "shopping" at our Halloween Store. At the "store," all their favorite healthy snacks can be bought for a price—six pieces of candy, eight pieces, and so on. Other items such as note pads and crayons can also be purchased. With this modification, our daughters can still have fun on Halloween acquiring lots of candy—but now they don't have to suffer the consequences of eating it. (Note: After debating the cost and fruitlessness of our household handing out organic candy only to have it be lost among all the other sugar goodies, we still decided that we simply could not pass out traditional candy and support the sugar industry with such a purchase. We give out organic candy, sweetened only with rice syrup.)

CHRISTMAS—The chances of Santa passing out rice crackers instead of candy canes are just about nil. But to question any action of Santa is to tread on shaky ground. Even my eldest pointed out that since Santa "knows everything," he should know not to give them anything with sugar. We have gotten around the "Santa issue" by having him write our girls at the beginning of the Christmas season. The letter explains how Santa (in his infinite wisdom) is quite aware that our girls do not eat sugar, but that he is also aware that most other children have not yet learned about the hazards of sugar and might not understand if Santa gave them some other kind of treat. Santa tells the girls that when they see him, he will still give them the sugar treat—however, they are to watch for his wink. That wink will be his little signal that they should trade in the sugar treat for a healthy one at home. Throughout the holiday season, as my girls sit upon various Santa laps, it is not difficult to request (with camera in hand), "How about a little wink, Santa?" And, on Christmas Eve, there was no question as to what to leave for Santa by the tree—he would of course be delighted to receive an organic oatmeal raisin cookie and a glass of almond milk for a nice, healthy change.

BIRTHDAY PARTIES—We have pointed out to our children that, hope-fully, the reason they are attending a friend's birthday party is not just for the cake and ice cream. Rather, we stress that they have been invited to help celebrate their friend's special day. Since our children agree, we offer them an alternative to eating the traditional birthday foods. We simply supply them with their own piece of organic cake to eat while the other guests eat the party cake. As for the ice cream (which, admittedly, is a little more diffi-cult to pack), we tell them that if they forgo eating ice cream at the party, they can then "trade it in" for some non-dairy ice cream when they get home.

IMPROVING TAP WATER

Along with all the dietary changes thus mentioned, it may also be neces-sary for individuals to improve the quality of the water they use in their home. Different water purifying systems are available, and each system does something a little different. The three main types of systems are reverse os-mosis (water molecules are forced through a semipermeable membrane while charred particles and larger molecules are repelled), distillation (water is boiled, converted to steam, and then condensed; whatever won't boil or evaporate is left behind), and active carbon filtration (water is passed through carbon that captures the contaminants).

Carbon filters, usually the least expensive of the three systems, are very effective for removing chlorine, organic chemicals and pesticides. A carbon filter will not, however, remove fluoride, salts, minerals, or nitrates. Reverse osmosis will remove all of these contaminants. However, Debra Dadd, au-thor of *Nontoxic and Natural*, advises that due to the amount of plastic used in the reverse osmosis system (that could potentially leach into the water), this water should not be used for drinking unless it is additionally purified with carbon filtration. Distillation will usually not remove light-molecule, volatile organic compounds. Some other disadvantages of distilla-tion are that the boiling chamber must be cleaned frequently and that it takes a significant amount of time to purify small quantities of water.

Testing the water of your home (see Appendix 2) will help you deter-mine which system will be the most beneficial for purifying it. Systems can then be put into an entire house or can be bought as units designed to filter individual faucets. Typically, individual units are placed in the kitchen to ensure an endless supply of pure water for drinking, washing produce, and cooking with. (I've always thought it was taking one step forward and two steps backward for people to buy organic vegetables but wash them in toxic water.)

Keep in mind that whatever toxins are in your tap water, that you are avoiding by not drinking it, can also be absorbed through your skin when you shower and bathe. According to the *American Journal of Public Health*, more toxins enter a body through bathing in toxic water than by drinking toxic water.

In our home, we decided to install an activated charcoal unit, which purifies the water coming out of every faucet in the house. The unit we bought has a thirty gallon tank and looks somewhat similar to a water softening unit. One of the features that we were specifically looking for, which this unit has, is "backflushing." Backflushing is when the water runs backwards through the carbon filter to clean it. Our unit backflushes once every six days. With this feature, we never have to worry about changing the carbon filter. I cannot even begin to write how great it is to have filtered water coming out of every faucet in my home.

I realize that since water purifying systems can be expensive, not everyone will be able to rush out and buy one today. However, there are a few things you can do to reduce the toxins in your water that do not cost anything. First, water can be boiled in a glass pot for ten minutes and then allowed to cool until the steaming stops. This is effective for removing chlorine, chlorine by-products, pesticides, and killing bacteria, but it will not remove organic chemicals, heavy metals, or trace minerals. Also, run cold water through each faucet in the home for at least ten minutes before drinking it if the water has not been turned on within the past six hours. (While this tactic may reduce contamination, it is not ideal from a conservation perspective or even feasible in areas suffering from a water shortage.)

Eliminating Lead from School Drinking Water

The Safe Drinking Water Act (SDWA) of 1974 required the EPA to set safe drinking water standards for the public. A 1986 amendment to the SDWA bans the use of lead materials in new plumbing and in plumbing repairs. This amendment also requires water suppliers to notify the public about lead in drinking water. In 1988, the Lead Contamination Control Act, another major amendment to the SDWA, became law.

The 1988 amendment spells out the specific guidelines for testing, recalling, repairing, and/or replacing water coolers that have parts containing lead or lead lined storage tanks. The amendment also outlines civil and criminal penalties for the manufacture and sale of water coolers containing lead. Last of all, the amendment authorizes grants to states to help them enforce the specifications of this law.

Fortunately, parents can now refer to the Lead Contamination Control

Act to insist that school officials take responsibility for the quality of the water in their schools. Parents can form a committee with other concerned individuals to inform other parents, teachers, and school administrators of the problem of lead contamination in school drinking water. The committee can first check to see if the school is abiding by the lead ban that states were required to adopt by June 1988 as part of the 1986 amendment to the SDWA. This can be done by checking with the state's department of health or by checking to see if plumbers or contractors who are making additions or repairs to the plumbing are using only lead-free materials. According to the SDWA, solder and flux are considered lead-free if they contain not more than 0.2 percent lead (in the past, solder was approximately 50 percent lead). Pipes as well as pipe fittings are now considered to be lead-free if they contain no more than 8 percent lead.

The committee can also request that school districts supply parents with the answers to a questionnaire developed by the EPA (see Appendix 5). This survey is designed to develop a specific plumbing profile for each individual school.

A government booklet, "Lead in School Drinking Water," provides good information about lead in school drinking water. This comprehensive manual can be purchased from the Superintendent of Documents, U.S. Printing Office, Washington, DC 20402. Written in a format that is easy to understand, the booklet explains in detail how to interpret the school plumbing profile, how to go about getting your school's water tested, how to interpret the results, and how to implement permanent solutions.

While changes are being implemented, school water systems can be flushed (details for how to do this effectively are included in the booklet) by maintenance personnel before classes begin each day; however, one disadvantage of flushing is the amount of water it uses (as already noted). Other steps that can be immediately implemented to reduce lead levels include frequently cleaning debris from all accessible screens and using only cold water for the preparation of food and beverages in the school cafeteria (hot water dissolves lead more readily than cold).

Every time it seems too overwhelming to try to influence your child's school district to do something about the water, a visit to the school might motivate you. Just stand on the playground during recess and count how many children drink water from the fountains. It is my hope that every parent would want to have documented proof that the water their children are drinking at school is safe by at least EPA's standards.

IN THE FUTURE

Unquestionably, both the average citizen and the traditional medical society are beginning to notice an undeniable link between diet and health. Countless articles in numerous magazines have addressed this topic. Likewise, many product labels now boast claims such as "cholesterol free" and "100% natural," indications that even the food industry acknowledges that people want to eat healthier food.

Recently, a healthy diet was the focus of a most unusual sentence for a young man in Britain who had numerous convictions for burglary. In lieu of a jail sentence, the seventeen-year-old was given the alternative of replacing his junk food diet with healthier food (whole grains, fresh vegetables and fruit) and taking a multi-vitamin and zinc. Weeks later, the boy was described as turning from a compulsive delinquent into a model citizen.

The youth's unusual sentence is part of a radical idea in Cumbria (northwest England), where the magistrates in juvenile courts have agreed to test the theory that antisocial behavior may be triggered by diet and toxins in the environment. Superintendent Peter Bennet of the West Yorkshire police in the north of England is currently preparing a project in which all juvenile offenders will be required to undergo nutritional testing before appearing in court. Once Bennet's program is set up, the results will be analyzed by the food and nutrition unit at Bradford University.

I get encouraged when I read about such events. Even though I personally have experienced the positive effects of eating a balanced diet instead of the traditional standard American diet (sometimes referred to as S.A.D.), I know that the masses have yet to experience this for themselves. So, I become encouraged when I hear about innovative programs which may not only help youngsters, but which also might enlighten others about the powerful effect a healthy diet can have on us.

I am also encouraged that changes in diet will occur because I firmly believe that parents *do* want to give their children the best food available. It's okay to feel overwhelmed by the challenge; I can certainly remember feeling that way myself. But please remember, somewhere between the Oreos and the tofu, I promise the obstacles and difficulties will lessen and the rewards will increase.

CHECKLIST FOR SUGGESTED CHANGES AND COMMITMENTS

☐ Avoid fast food restaurants.

☐ If meat and poultry remain in your diet, buy only organic meat and poultry, that does not contain antibiotics, growth hormones, or pesticide residues.

☐ To guard against salmonella poisoning, pack raw meat and poultry separately to keep them from dripping on other groceries, In addition, raw meat and poultry should be refrigerated as soon as possible, thawed in the refrigerator (as opposed to at room temperature), and cooked thoroughly. Also wash hands and utensils immediately after handling raw meat or poultry.

☐ Substitute soy "cold cuts" for meat and poultry factory leftovers.

☐ Eat only deep-water fish.

☐ Locate a local health food store or mail-order company to purchase items not typically found in local grocery stores.

☐ Begin replacing sugar goodies with treats made with rice syrup, barley malt, or fruit.

☐ Substitute fruit-sweetened cereal or cereal made with rice syrup or barley malt for sugar-sweetened cereals.

☐ Eliminate all foods that contain artificial colors.

☐ Do not purchase food in lead-soldered cans. (Lead cans have crimped seams in an irregular line of silver-gray metal along the joint.)

☐ Replace all teflon and aluminum cookware since they can contaminate food.

☐ Scrutinize food labels and avoid buying food containing additives and preservatives which have been the subject of concern.

☐ Eat organic whole grains (e.g., rice, barley, oats, rye).

☐ Eat organic beans (e.g., navy, kidney, soy, lentil).

☐ Buy only organically grown produce (or at least produce that is grown domestically).

☐ Purchase processed foods made with organic ingredients.

☐ Substitute sea salt for refined salt.

☐ Begin to eliminate dairy products.

☐ Use soy or almond milk in recipes requiring milk.

☐ Substitute soy cheese for dairy cheese.

☐ Substitute ice cream made from soy or rice for dairy ice cream.

☐ Buy and drink purified water in glass rather than plastic containers since plastic can leach into the water.

☐ Purchase a water purifying system.

☐ Begin reading books about cooking "whole foods."

☐ Enroll in a "whole foods" cooking class.

☐ Try a modified or structured "traditional whole foods" diet for at least six months, and then evaluate you family's health and general well-being. (Remember, there is no one diet that is right for everyone since each of us is unique. The premise of a whole foods diet, whether implemented fully or not, can serve as an effective guideline for any future diet.)

☐ Organize a committee to ensure that the drinking water at your children's school is safe.

Quiz 5—A Pretest on Reproductive Function

1. The March of Dimes estimates that of the approximate 250,000 American babies born each year with defects, _____ percent of the defects are caused by food additives, environmental pollutants, drugs, and alcohol.[1]
   A) 10
   B) 50
   C) 80

2. Lead has been known to interfere with reproductive function since _____.
   A) Ancient Rome
   B) the Industrial Revolution
   C) the turn of the century

3. In a study of ten teratogenic compounds, humans were actually found to be more susceptible *at lower doses* than the most sensitive animals tested for _____ of the compounds.
   A) three
   B) eight
   C) nine

4. According to a report published by the *American Journal of Epidemiology*, children whose mothers slept under electric blankets during the first trimester of pregnancy have a _____ greater chance of developing a brain tumor.
   A) two times
   B) four times
   C) ten times

5. In a case control study done to determine the causes of leukemia in children ten years and younger, the study showed an increased risk for children whose *fathers* had been exposed to chlorinated solvents at work _____.
   A) prior to the child's birth
   B) after the child's birth

6. "Fetal protection policies" _____.
   A) protect pregnant women from chemical exposures while at work.
   B) provide employees with a compensated leave of absence while pregnant
   C) deny employment to fertile and/or pregnant women who may be exposed to hazardous chemicals on the job

Answers to Reproductive Function Quiz

1. C While some birth defects are caused by mutations (genetically inherited), others are caused by chemical agents which cause changes in the developing fetus. Pregnant women may be exposed to these chemicals without even knowing it.

2. A Even though lead has been known to interfere with reproductive function since Ancient Rome, it is still adversely affecting some pregnant women and their fetuses in modern times. Exposures to lead can cause spontaneous abortions and stillbirths; prenatal exposures can cause learning disabilities, brain damage, and mental retardation.

3. B Many individuals believe that *animal* studies indicating toxicity have no bearing on human health. However, with some chemicals, humans experience adverse health effects at *lower* doses than test animals.

4. B Many researchers now believe that electromagnetic fields are associated with cancer. While high-power transmission lines have been implicated, many studies now show that home electrical items, such as electric blankets, may also be hazardous. The reasons the risks of cancer may be higher with an electric blanket as opposed to other home electrical appliances is because of the close proximity between the field and the person and because the exposure is usually extended (all night).

5. B The children and spouses of persons working with toxic chemicals can also be exposed to the chemicals when the person carries residues of the chemicals home on work clothing and equipment.

6. C Currently, "fetal protection policies" apply to women but not men. This policy has been questioned since many of the chemicals that are considered too hazardous for women to work with have also proven to be equally hazardous to the male reproductive system. To date, at least five discrimination suits have been filed against companies during the last ten years, but no legal precedent has been established.

CHAPTER FIVE

Our Babies: Before and After

The due date for the birth of my second daughter was April 16. As March approached, I was not concerned that I had still not sorted the baby items, set up the crib, or organized some kind of sane schedule for the rest of my family to follow. After all, I still had plenty of time.

However, to our great surprise, Kiley was born on *March 4*, six weeks early. Our premature daughter entered the world weighing a mere four and a half pounds.

At the time, our daughter's early birth baffled us—especially since our first daughter had been born right on time. But now, two and a half years (and some miles of wisdom) later, we are no longer surprised that Kiley was born prematurely.

Kiley was conceived two months after we moved into a brand new home—the same home which we now know was continually outgassing toxic carpet, paint, and furniture vapors. While I was pregnant, our home was sprayed five times by our pest control service.

These facts now seem so relevant in retrospect. However, back then, we never considered any of these environmental factors as possible reasons for our daughter's premature birth.

At the detox clinic, I remember being surprised to meet several other patients who had also given birth to premature babies. There seemed to be some kind of correlation, but, at the time, I still did not know what it might be.

While researching this book, the connection became quite obvious. I was amazed at the number of articles and studies I uncovered—some of which had been conducted several decades ago—that focused on the effects chemical exposures can have on reproductive function. Not only did these reports suggest the possible link between toxins and premature births, but they also cited the effects of toxins on other reproductive functions.

No, I cannot scientifically prove that Kiley was premature because of my continual toxic exposures. Babies are premature for a wide variety of reasons. But, I truly believe that Kiley's early arrival was due to the endless chemicals to which I had exposed both myself and my unborn baby.

Whether or not this was the case, the fact remains that there *is* documented proof that toxins can adversely affect the reproductive system. Exposure to hazardous chemicals can cause miscarriage, premature births, stillbirths, birth defects, and the occurrence of cancer some time later in the child's life.

Most likely, the information in this chapter will be new to parents. It is not usually discussed at childbirth classes, play groups, or PTA meetings. Likewise, it is not usually discussed with your obstetrician or pediatrician. I knew almost nothing about chemicals and reproductive function prior to or during either of my two pregnancies. Certainly, I thought of many things while I was pregnant—but I honestly do not recall ever thinking about whether or not pesticides or formaldehyde were harming my unborn baby. No one ever warned me about the hazards associated with common household cleaning chemicals, leaded gasoline, or the chemicals my husband was exposed to at his work, for example.

I now find it rather ironic that when I was pregnant I would suffer through a severe cold without indulging in even one cold medication because I was concerned about its impact on the baby. However, at the same time, I was living in a new home that was outgassing a variety of toxic chemicals and was repeatedly being sprayed with pesticides.

This chapter focuses on the effects toxins can have on babies both *before* and *after* they are born. It describes the effects of toxins on the reproductive systems of both males and females, how and which chemicals can directly affect the fetus in the mother's womb, and the dangers of being exposed to chemicals at work. The chapter also addresses how children are exposed to toxins every day after they are born, beginning with breast milk contamination.

Most parents hope that they are providing the best for their children. I know we did. To believe that we may be poisoning our children sounds more like something out of a Stephen King novel. But, unfortunately, it may be true. Our children now live in a chemical world unlike anything we were ever exposed to as infants. Therefore, I believe it is imperative that prospective parents understand how chemicals can directly affect their children and their unborn children, because, as with everything else in parenting, we often don't get a second chance.

THE PROBLEMS

TOXINS THAT CAN AFFECT REPRODUCTIVE FUNCTION AND OFFSPRING

Teratogens

A teratogen is a chemical substance that adversely affects the embryo at doses below those necessary to produce overt signs of toxicity in pregnant women. After conception, exposures to teratogenic substances have been known to cause miscarriages, stillbirths, low birth weights, and birth defects.

Probably the most publicized example of a teratogen is the drug Thalidomide, which was given to women in the 1960s as a "safe tranquilizer." While Thalidomide had no apparent toxic effect on pregnant women, the babies of mothers who took the drug were often born with malformed arms and legs.

Humans have proven to be *more* sensitive to the teratogenic effects of the drug than animals. For example, humans are sixty times more sensitive than rats, two hundred times more sensitive than dogs, and *seven hundred* times more sensitive than hamsters.[2]

After significant numbers of deformed babies were born to mothers who had taken Thalidomide, the medical profession was forced to back down on its original stand that the placenta can prevent harmful bacteria and toxic chemicals from reaching the fetus. Doctors had previously thought that only German Measles and syphilis could pass through the placenta and harm a fetus.

Today, it is known that the placenta can prevent *some* substances from reaching the fetus. However, other substances can pass through easily. According to Dr. Arthur J. Vadar, "almost all environmental chemicals which can make it into the mother's bloodstream, will pass, to a lesser or greater extent, into the fetus."

The toxic substances can affect the fetus in a variety of ways. For example, lead can concentrate in the brain of the embryo and subsequently cause brain damage, whereas pesticides can accumulate in fetal fat and later cause mental disorders or organ damage.

Other variables also determine whether or not a teratogen will affect the fetus. These include the gestational age at which the exposure occurred, the dose of the exposure, the route in which the chemical entered the pregnant woman, and the actual genetic make-up of the unborn child. The final effect upon a child can vary from none to even a fatal outcome.

Thus far, my youngest daughter is an example of the unpredictable effects of toxins. While I still cannot tell you if the chemical burden Kiley inherited will ultimately affect her health (since many of the effects of these chemicals take years to manifest themselves), I can tell you that, so far, she is strong and healthy, and has been since birth. In fact, hours before her arrival into this world, I was informed that she was going to have to be rushed by ambulance to the children's hospital because testing showed that her lungs were not yet mature. But even back then, she defied the norm—to everyone's surprise her breathing was absolutely fine when she was born.

I obviously hope that she will continue to defy the odds and will not develop any adverse health effects in the future as the result of her past exposures to chemicals. It is possible that she will continue to be healthy. Without question, not every fetus exposed to a teratogen is affected. However, I now consider exposing oneself while pregnant to known or suspected teratogens is equivalent to playing Russian Roulette with a fetus.

According to the late Dr. Phyllis Saifer, a leading expert in this field, there is evidence that indicates that the following medications and chemicals may damage a fetus:

- *anticancer drugs*, drugs designed to kill malignant cells may also kill healthy cells in the embryo
- *anticoagulants*, may cause facial and optical defects, mental retardation, and other central nervous system abnormalities
- *anti-infection drugs*, may cause liver dysfunction
- *tetracycline*, has been known to cause tooth discoloration in infants
- *anti-inflammatory agents*, may adversely affect the fetal cardiovascular system
- *antipsychotic drugs*, may cause jaundice and muscle tremors in newborns.
- *hormones*, may cause fetal heart defects
- *tranquilizers*, associated with congenital malformations and breathing problems in newborns

Of course, in all cases, a pregnant woman must determine if the benefits of taking a particular medication outweigh the known risks to the fetus.

In addition, Dr. Saifer warns that the following metals and chemicals are teratogens and may also be harmful to a fetus: arsenic, cadmium, gold, lead, mercury, acrylonitrile, aldicarb, benzene, chlordane, dioxin, ethylene dibromide, polychlorinated biphenyls (PCBs), BHT, EDTA, PVP, DBCP, toluene, and vinyl chloride. Unfortunately, these chemicals can be found in products and in commercial, home, and work environments which pregnant women come in contact with daily. For example, BHT, EDTA, and PVP are commonly found in food and cosmetics; vinyl chloride is a popular plastic used to make countless everyday products, including furniture, car interiors, and toys; benzene is found in paints, solvents, glues, and cleaning fluids; and toluene is found in nail polish, spot removers, and permanent marking pens.

Mutagens

Mutagens are chemicals that cause gene mutations. Mutations occur when the DNA of the sperm or egg is altered, subsequently changing the genetic coding for future generations. This change in the DNA can result in one of two adverse effects. First, the change in the genetic code may prevent successful fertilization from ever taking place because the DNA no longer matches the template for reproduction (i.e., sterility). Second, the change in the genetic code may trigger hereditary diseases and/or congenital malformations.

Assessing the effects of toxic chemical exposures becomes very complicated when we consider that the adverse effect of a mutagen might not become manifested until future generations. For example, a woman may be exposed to a chemical in her twenties without any apparent effect. However, this exposure may be responsible for later causing a birth defect in her *grandchild*. Evaluating the adverse effects of toxic exposures becomes even further complicated when we consider how difficult it would be to determine *which* of the woman's past chemical exposures was specifically responsible for the birth defect. Her multiple past chemical exposures and the extended time period between exposure and effect would make it almost impossible to determine which chemical had triggered the birth defect. However, not being able to prove which mutagen caused a birth defect does not mean that mutagens do not exist or that we cannot be exposed to them.

It always frightens me when I think about mutagens. The existence of such chemicals in our daily lives makes it impossible for us to really know the effect our daily exposures to chemicals are having upon our families.

Effects of Toxins on the Male Reproductive System

In addition to affecting DNA coding, toxic chemicals can affect all aspects of the reproductive system—not just during pregnancy and *not just the reproductive system of women.* Exposure to toxic chemicals can affect a couple's plans to start a family by impairing male sperm production.

In 1980, Friends of the Earth published the shocking results of its comparison of thirty-two studies on male fertility, conducted between 1929 and 1979. These studies included both American and European males, many of whom where randomly selected. The results showed that in 1930 the average male sperm count was 120 million(M) per milliliter(ml) compared to less than 80 M/ml just two generations later. The more recent studies show average male sperm count to be 20 M/ml. A male with a sperm count this low is considered functionally sterile, meaning that conception is difficult. The average sperm count has fallen off so dramatically, that in 1980 it was estimated that *20 percent* of all American males were functionally sterile.[3] Many researchers have implicated the increased use of chemicals, such as pesticides, and heavy metals, which have been documented to interfere with normal sperm production, as the reason for such a dramatic change in sperm count. Dr. Ralph Dougherty, a leading expert in this field, attributes increased sterility to chlorinated hydrocarbons, particularly PCBs, in our environment.

Functional sterility does not just apply to older men either. A study done at major American universities showed that *25 percent of today's college students are sterile*. Thirty-five years ago less than 0.5 percent were sterile.[4]

Sterility among males is so high that major sperm banks are having problems finding acceptable donors. According to John Olson, director of one of the oldest commercial private sperm banks in the United States, it never used to be a problem finding high quality semen donors. Olson states that now his sperm bank has to reject *nine out of ten applicants*.[5]

Considering the amount of toxic chemicals in our lives today, it is likely that the numbers of functionally sterile men will continue to rise. The implications of this are staggering. Does this mean that as many as 50 percent of the young male children today will be sterile adults, and as many as 75 percent of the next generation? How high must this percentage be before we finally accept that daily chemicals can adversely affect reproductive function? For those friends of mine who continue to spray pesticides in and around their homes, I often wonder if their children (as possible sterile adults) will concur that it was indeed better to eliminate the ants in the kitchen with toxic pesticides rather than try a nontoxic alternative. Moreover, I wonder how understanding these young adults will be if they discover that their parents *knew* of the overwhelming information linking pesticides and sterility but chose to use pesticides anyway.

That exposures to pesticides can cause sterility is nothing new. Back in the 1970s, an infamous incident involving workers in a chemical plant in California that manufactured the pesticide DBCP clearly demonstrated how male reproductive function may be affected by exposures to pesticides. At this plant, there were several young married men anxious to begin families. However, strangely, after a considerable period of time none of the wives of these men had become pregnant.

In 1977, after medical testing, the reason became clear. It turned out that the men exhibited both atrophy of the testicles and decreased sperm production as a result of their exposure to DBCP at the plant. The tests also showed that each of the men produced an unusually high number of abnormal sperm. The final prognosis was that the men were sterile. (DBCP has now also been classified as a carcinogen.)

Since then, other toxins have also been proven to affect male reproductive function. At the American Cyanamid Company, female employees had to undergo voluntary sterilization if they wanted to keep their jobs when it became known that their exposures to lead might affect pregnancies. (The company was afraid of lawsuits.) However, it was later determined by OSHA (Occupational Safety and Health Administration) that the levels of lead at the plant were equally dangerous to the male employees.

In males, exposures to toxins not only affect fertility, but can also subsequently affect the health of the fetus. There are two theories as to how this can happen. One theory is that toxins directly damage the genetic coding in sperm since toxins can collect and concentrate in the male reproductive tract. The second theory is that toxins are carried in the semen during intercourse that occurs after conception. It is thought that the semen is then absorbed through the vaginal walls and enters the blood flowing to the fetus. Either of these two theories may explain why so many Vietnam War veterans who were involved in the use of Agent Orange have had children with birth defects. It may also explain why a study done at the University of Southern California found a definite correlation between fathers exposed to toxic chemicals and children having brain tumors.

CHEMICAL EXPOSURES AT WORK THAT CAN AFFECT REPRODUCTIVE FUNCTION AND OFFSPRING

The United States government estimates that between fifteen to twenty million jobs in this country expose employees to some type of reproductive hazard. The actual effects will vary with the type of chemical(s) used on the job. For example, male workers exposed to metals such as mercury, lead, cadmium, arsenic, and zinc have suffered chromosome damage, while their wives have had a significantly higher number of miscarriages. It is not clear if these metals actually damage sperm, which then results in an abnormal fetus, or if the women become contaminated when the men carry the metals into their homes via work clothing and equipment.

Since ancient times, lead has been recognized as a metal that interferes with reproductive function. In females, exposures to lead have been known to cause menstrual disorders, infertility, spontaneous abortions, and still-births. Prenatal exposures to lead are equally hazardous. Learning disabilities, brain damage and mental retardation can be caused by even small intrauterine exposures to lead.

It is important to note that approximately 90 percent of the lead that enters the atmosphere comes from the combustion of gasoline. Therefore, everyone, not just those persons who are employed as battery manufacturers, painters, typesetters, or stained glass artists, are routinely exposed to lead (see chapter 4 for a more in-depth discussion of the effects of lead).

Exposures to many other substances at work have also been known to adversely affect reproductive function. For example, artists, potters, glass blowers, and people who manufacture varnishes, inks, rubber, and wood preservatives are exposed to manganese dust, which may cause impotence or other sexual dysfunction. Vinyl chloride, considered a mutagen, is used in the manufacturing of plastic and can cause sexual difficulties, miscarriages, and possible birth defects. Formaldehyde, to which more than two million United States workers are exposed, may cause low sperm count, menstrual problems, and anemia during pregnancy. Likewise, carbon disulfide, a fumigant used in the manufacturing of rayon, is known to impair semen quality and reduce the size of testicles.

Ironically, chemicals used by health professionals pose some of the greatest reproductive hazards. For example, pregnant women who are exposed to ethylene oxide, which is used to sterilize objects, risk damage to the DNA of their unborn child since ethylene oxide is a mutagen. In addition, pregnant women handling ethylene oxide have a higher risk of miscarriage. Chronic exposures to various anesthetic gases have been linked to infertility in men, increased rates of spontaneous abortions, and low birth rates. Studies have also shown an increased rate of birth defects in babies born to hospital personnel who worked with anesthetic gases prior to and during pregnancy.

Here's a list of other occupations and some of the hazardous toxins associated with each:

- *Aircraft workers*, chlorinated solvents, hydraulic fluids, welding fumes, and radiation.

- *Carpenters and construction workers*, adhesives, paints, asbestos fibers, insulation, plastics, solvents, and varnishes.

- *Dry cleaning employees*, ethylene dibromide (for waterproofing and protective finishings) and naphthalene (for mothproofing).

- *Electricians*, PCBs (in insulation), radiation (in appliances), and cadmium (in solder).

- *Farmers and agriculture workers*, fungicides, pesticides, herbicides, and ethylene gas (used to accelerate ripening).

- *Fumigators*, fungicides, pesticides, herbicides, benzene, chloroform, formaldehyde, lindane, propane and other propellants.

- *Furniture makers*, formaldehyde, lacquer solvents, pentachlorophenol, varnishes, and stains.

- *Jewelers*, lacquer solvents, lead, mercury, benzene, and arsenic fumes.

- *Printers*, benzene, formaldehyde, lead (in wallpaper printing), toluene, and xylene.

- *Photographers*, ammonia (in automatic film processing), formaldehyde, chlorine, phenols, and sulfuric acid.

- *Plumbers*, asbestos, chloroform, lye, and polyurethane

The list goes on. Currently, a significant number of specific chemicals are being studied for their effects on reproductive functions (see Appendix 7). These chemicals appear in a variety of workplaces and are also commonly found in the home.

BREAST MILK CONTAMINATION

When my premature daughter was born, she was too small to breast-feed successfully. Nonetheless, everyday I awakened at two in the morning and "bonded" with my electric pump to faithfully express my milk, which I then put into bottles made especially for premature babies. I was determined my daughter would have breast milk—even if her mouth was too small to breast-feed normally. When my milk supplied dried up a month later, I was heartbroken and concerned that my daughter was not going to get my "wonderful" milk. However, in view of what I have now learned about toxins in breast milk, I am not sure that I would have felt as badly about it today.

I now know that breast milk can become contaminated from toxic chemicals stored in a woman's body fat. According to the EPA, the average American breast-fed baby ingests nine times the permissible level of dieldrin, a potent, cancer-causing agent. Likewise, the EPA states that the average American breast-fed infant ingests ten times the FDA's maximum allowable intake of PCBs. (In doses as low as a few parts per billion, PCBs can cause birth defects and cancer in test animals).

Moreover, even though DDT was banned in 1972 because of its known toxicity, a current study shows no decrease in the amount of DDT in breast milk. This fact not only suggests that past chemical exposures remain in the body for long periods of time, but, I believe, also confirms reports that DDT is still commonly used as a secret inert ingredient in some pesticides. The study states that a substantial percentage of nursing infants are ingesting more DDT than is considered acceptable.[6] In fact, it was pointed out that cow's milk containing equivalent amounts of DDT would be banned by the FDA.

Breast milk becomes contaminated because during lactation body fat mobilization is increased and toxins which have been stored in the fat are released into the bloodstream. The more toxins the nursing mother has been exposed to in her life the more probable it is that her milk will be contaminated.

However, the American Academy of Pediatrics currently states that there is no evidence to suggest that the levels of contaminants found in mother's milk are actually dangerous to nursing infants. Yet, when I read such a statement, I cannot help but recall my own past experiences with reputable doctors who also did not believe that my chemical exposures were harming me. Moreover, there are other scientists and doctors who have conducted their own studies and do not agree with the Academy's conclusion. These other studies suggest that *premature* infants may be more affected by contaminated breast milk, because premature babies tend to have impaired elimination mechanisms and their blood-brain barrier may be more easily breached. This latter fact is especially significant since pesticides and their solvent materials are *neurotoxins* and since substantial brain maturation occurs *after birth*.

These disturbing facts about breast milk do not, however, automatically imply that cow's milk is the safer alternative. In a sampling of cow's milk, the following residues were detected: 96 percent contained dieldrin, 93 percent contained heptachlor epoxide, 73 percent contained lindane, 69 percent contained chlordane, and 48 percent contained DDT.[7] Formula can also be contaminated with toxic chemicals.

Too much evidence still supports breast milk *as the best nutritional choice for a young infant.* Not only does nature ensure that breast milk contains all the nutrients necessary for a baby, but the milk also contains antibodies that are crucial to a newborn. Likewise, breast-feeding can be an opportunity for a wonderful, emotional bonding between a mother and child. However, breast-feeding mothers should be aware of the possibility of breast milk contamination and should take certain precautions (discussed in the solutions section of this chapter) to protect their baby.

BABY CARE PRODUCTS

I think it's extremely important to point out that many of the toxic chemicals discussed in the book thus far can also be found in countless commercial baby products on the market today. Many baby care products used to soothe or clean an infant's skin typically contain BHA /BHT, fragrance and talc. BHA is a suspected human carcinogen. In animal studies, both BHA and BHT were shown to cause metabolic stress, depression of growth rate, liver damage, weight loss, baldness, and fetal abnormalities. The word "fragrance" on a baby product label can refer to up to 4,000 different ingredients, none of which are usually listed on the label. Most fragrances are synthetic and have been noted to cause numerous types of central nervous system symptoms in clinical observations.

Even something as basic as baby powder may be very harmful. Talc, an ingredient in most baby powders, may be contaminated with carcinogenic asbestos. Talc baby powders can also be hazardous if accidentally inhaled or ingested. Approximately fifty cases of baby powder inhalation are reported to the New York Poison Control Center each year. When talc is inhaled, a baby may develop severe, acute, or chronic respiratory conditions; when the exposure is massive (by accidental aspiration), death may even occur. In a report of twenty-five cases of talcum powder aspiration, 20 percent of the children died. Dr. Barry H. Rumack of the Rocky Mountain Poison Center believes that talcum powder should be completely removed from a child's environment.

Disposable Diapers

While researching information for this book, I had the opportunity to change the diaper of a friend's child. This was my first exposure to disposable diapers since becoming chemically sensitive. As I went about completing this trivial task, I was amazed at the overwhelming chemical odors coming from the diaper. In just the short time it took to diaper the child, my eyelids had swelled, and I had gotten a headache. I remembered all those countless disposable diapers we had used on our own girls' cute derrieres. Suddenly, I found myself wondering why I had never really thought about just *what* had kept their bottoms dry.

After all, we knew that our daughters typically urinated several times before the diaper needed changing. But just how did I think my children remained dry? Did I think some magical diaper fairy whisked away urine with her magic wand? Of course not. But did I ever internalize that *chemicals* were keeping my babies dry? Probably not.

Disposable diapers contain numerous chemicals. Dyes, fragrances, acrylics, polyester, and polyethylene are all chemicals found in such diapers, which are snugly placed around Baby round-the-clock for the first two or more years of his or her life. (It is estimated that a baby spends approximately 20,000 hours in diapers.) Dyes have been known to cause anemia, as well as damage to the central nervous system, kidneys, and liver. According to the FDA, fragrances can cause headaches, dizziness, and rashes. Polyethylene is a suspected human carcinogen.

In addition to trapping wetness, plastic disposable diapers also trap warmth. The temperature inside a disposable diaper can be as high as 104 degrees. These hot and sticky conditions create a perfect environment for bacteria to grow in.

In a study of one-month-old infants, 54 percent of the infants who were wearing disposable diapers had rashes and 16 percent had severe rashes. However, only 18 percent of the infants who were wearing cloth diapers had rashes; none had severe rashes.[8] Some possible reasons for the increased rate of diaper rash among disposable diaper wearers are that some infants may be allergic to the chemicals in the diapers, disposable diapers are changed less often since they feel dry on the outside, and disposable diapers reduce air circulation and increase temperature.

Another concern with disposable diapers that has received a considerable amount of media attention lately is the impact disposable diapers have and will have on the environment. In 1989, *sixteen billion* used diapers went into landfills, and two billion more were incinerated. Aside from the important general concern that our landfills are already filled to capacity, there is the concern that soiled diapers stored underground may contaminate our ground water. In addition, it is *not* true that some disposable diapers are biodegradable. "Biodegradable" diapers simply have had cornstarch added to them during the manufacturing process. Cornstarch aids in breaking diapers apart, but it does not enable the diaper to actually biodegrade.

After learning about the chemicals in disposable diapers, one day at the store I found myself staring at the words "chemical-free" printed on the packages of several brands of disposable diapers. The manufacturer of one brand was so confident of the product's claim that a toll-free number was printed on the package for consumers to call if they had any questions. I could not resist. Even though I didn't need any diapers, I purchased a package.

Before calling the company, I first put the diapers through a very unsophisticated, but completely reliable, chemical test—my nose. To the company's credit, when I pulled out the first diaper, I smelled practically nothing. Only the tape used to secure the diaper seemed to give off a distinct odor. I even risked several deep whiffs (something I would never have done with other diapers), but the diaper did not cause any reactions in me.

While I was willing to concede that these diapers did not contain as many chemicals as other brands, I still could not understand how the company could call them "chemical-free." After all, I was fairly confident that they had been chlorine-bleached (which meant they were probably not dioxin-free). I was also pretty sure that these diapers were made out of plastic. Furthermore, I seriously doubted that the colorful little whales and birdies gracing the top of the diaper had been hand painted with nontoxic watercolors.

I called the diaper manufacturer to confirm my suspicion that the diapers were not really chemical-free. At first, the representatives of the company were very cordial. They told me that, yes, the outer layers of "biodegradable" diapers are a mixture of cornstarch-based resin and plastic. When I pursued the point that if the company's diapers are made from plastic they could not be called chemical-free, I kept getting referred to other personnel. I did finally get an acknowledgement that the manufacturers of the diaper employed a chemical company to make this new "biodegradable plastic." When I asked if the biodegradable plastic had been tested for long- or short-term health effects, I was told yes; however, upon further questioning, I found out that all of the testing had been done by the company that made the plastic. Interestingly, my phone conversation also confirmed my "nose" test—the tape used to secure the diapers was made out of regular plastic.

When I once again expressed my confusion as to how this diaper could be called "chemical-free," the distraught representative on the other end of the phone grew somewhat indignant. Defending her company, she was quick to point out that it seemed to her that every time companies tried to do something good, someone always came along and criticized them. Her feeling was that her company's diaper was certainly an improvement over others. While she did not actually say it, she inferred that her company should be appreciated—not picked on.

I could see her point. Certainly, we want to encourage manufacturers to produce chemical-free products. But I would like to hold the applause until manufacturers truly start providing such products. I would not have had any qualms with this company if the diaper package had stated that the diapers contain fewer chemicals than other disposable diapers. But, the diapers are not "chemical-free," and to advertise it as such is unfair to concerned consumers, especially since these diapers cost approximately 30 percent more than other brands.

Toys

As my health slowly improves, I am becoming less sensitive to many chemicals. However, I will know that I am truly better when and if I can ever venture into a toy store. Ironically, the one store that still produces the most reactions in me is filled with products for *children*.

Without question, one reason that toy stores affect me is because so many toys are made out of vinyl plastic, including vinyl chloride, polyvinyl chloride (PVC), and polyvinylpyrrolidone (PVP). PVP is so hazardous that NASA has banned the use of it in space capsules. It is carcinogenic and can cause a lung disease called thesaurosis, in which enlarged lymph nodes, lung masses, and blood cell changes occur. PVC releases vinyl chloride, which is on the EPA's priority list of sixty-five pollutants recognized as being hazardous to human health. Vinyl chloride is carcinogenic, teratogenic, and mutagenic. It can cause numbness in the fingers, chronic bronchitis, and allergic reactions, as well as other adverse effects. Additionally, phthalic anhydride and other plasticizers used in PVC production can irritate the throat, mouth, and nose and burn the skin. Yet these materials are commonly used (with no printed warnings) in many toys designed for babies, toddlers, and older children.

Before I became aware that I am sensitive to plastics, I used to repeatedly remark how I always felt worse in our family room. We eventually made the "plastic" connection. After a quick glance around our family room back then, one might have easily mistaken the place for a toy showroom, since there was probably not a single plastic toy that my children did not own. Despite their bright colors and apparent appeal to children, these toys were outgassing chemicals that were unquestionably triggering adverse reactions in me. It still concerns me that I am so sensitive to products designed especially *for children*.

The Baby's Room

In addition to baby care products, diapers, and toys, other items found in a typical baby's room, especially if it was recently decorated, may also pose health problems. For example, crib mattresses may contain flame retardants, such as tetrakis hydroxylmethyl phosphonium (THPC). This common flame retardant releases formaldehyde when the fabric becomes wet.

Similarly, beds and bedding are often made from plastics that continually outgas harmful vapors. One such plastic, polyurethane, releases toluene diisoyanate, which can trigger serious pulmonary effects.

Sheets and pillowcases are often made from polyester, which in addition to being treated with formaldehyde, can cause eye and respiratory tract irritation and acute dermatitis. Likewise, cuddly baby blankets have probably been mothproofed with a pesticide and/or made from acrylic, nylon or polyester.

Furthermore, the walls of the nursery may have just been painted or wallpapered, the floor covered with new carpet, the room furnished with new furniture, and the closets filled with brand new polyester clothing (see chapter 3 for a discussion on the problems of outgassing).

Yet, it is to this very environment that a brand new infant is brought. It is in this environment that from the very first days of his or her life an infant must continually inhale outgassing toxic vapors. Moreover, it is not possible for an infant to tell a parent that these vapors are bothering him or her. The best an infant can do is cry, which has probably yet to be translated as "get me away from these toxic vapors!"

Sudden Infant Death Syndrome (SIDS)

As a new mother, I was terrified to learn that some infants just suddenly stop breathing and die. In fact, on several occasions, I woke my infant children from a sound sleep just to make sure that they were breathing. I also confess to breast-feeding my first daughter two months longer than I really wanted to because I had read of a slightly higher incidence of SIDS among bottle-fed babies. Frankly, I would have done just about anything if I thought it would decrease the possibility of SIDS.

The medical profession still cannot determine why these infants stop breathing. A recent preliminary study suggests that formaldehyde, which is present in just about every new baby item, may play a role in the death of these infants.[9] This theory does not seem far-fetched to me for the following reasons.

First, I know how formaldehyde affects my own breathing. In our old house, I would often awaken from a sound sleep completely horrified because I had stopped breathing for a few seconds. Interestingly, this has never happened in our new, nontoxic home.

Secondly, I have learned that children under the age of five breathe differently than adults. Because their respiratory tracts have fewer and narrower branches, younger children have a faster respiratory rate than adults. This means that young children are going to inhale more vapors in a room than an adult would in the same room. In addition, children tend to breathe more through their mouths, so a greater proportion of matter that would otherwise be trapped in the nasal passages will make its way to the child's lungs. These inhaled toxic substances can both injure lung tissue or be absorbed into the bloodstream and subsequently be transported to other parts of the body. Additionally, long-term exposures to toxic chemicals can impair the normal clearance mechanisms of the lung, thus increasing the possibility of tissue damage occurring when toxic material is inhaled.

Another reason I suspect a possible link between chemicals and SIDS is the documented higher incidence of SIDS in the wintertime. During the winter, windows are usually left closed, decreasing ventilation in every room, including the baby's room. Less ventilation increases the likelihood that outgassing vapors will be inhaled.

Finally, the mere fact that the traditional medical community cannot determine a cause for these horrible deaths makes me believe that SIDS may have a chemical connection. My own experience has repeatedly confirmed that the majority of traditional doctors have yet to acknowledge, let alone research, the adverse health effects of the countless chemicals in our lives.

FOULING THE NEST

"Fouling the nest" has become the phrase used to describe the unintentional contamination of one's home from exposures to chemicals or other substances at work. Fouling the nest often occurs when contaminated work clothing and/or work-related equipment is brought home each night. The people living in the home are then exposed to the toxic substances via inhalation and skin contact.

Exposure to asbestos at work is one example of "fouling the nest." Studies have shown that some family members of workers exposed to asbestos have developed asbestos-related diseases as much as thirty years later.[10] Interestingly, the wives of employees exposed to asbestos were most affected. This may be because the wives were the ones responsible for laundering their husband's work clothes or because they were in contact with their husbands for the longest amount of time.

Artists who work at home can also "foul the nest." Artists who have in-home studios and are self-employed are not monitored by the general regulations of the Occupational Safety and Health Administration (OSHA). Because their work environment is unregulated, some artists may believe that they are working under safe conditions. Unfortunately, this is often not the case.

Many art supplies are toxic. Yet, often the only warning that appears on an art product states "Use only in a well-ventilated area." However, this warning is too vague to be effective, because what is considered a well-ventilated area may vary greatly. For example, one artist may interpret this to mean one opened window, another may think it means two opened windows, a third may think it means three opened windows plus an exhaust fan. Considering that artists who work at home are daily exposing their families to toxic materials, this warning does not seem to be enough.

Furthermore, work environments that appear to have no negative impact on the health of adults may, in fact, be very hazardous for children. For example, while a New York couple who made stain glass in their kitchen noted no adverse health effects in themselves, their eighteen-month-old toddler was diagnosed as having lead poisoning as a result of exposure to the art materials that the parents used.

Hobby enthusiasts, regardless of their actual profession, may also be contaminating their homes. The Center for Safety in the Arts estimates that 100 million Americans, including children and hobbyists, are exposed to dangerous art materials without ever realizing it.

I, unfortunately, had the opportunity to meet a person who suffered severe reactions to the art supplies she used in her home. When I first met Barb, a painter, at the detox clinic, she was completely paralyzed from the waist down and in a wheelchair.

She had first started noticing some tingling in her feet and legs three years earlier. As time passed, these nerve sensations became worse. However, each time she went to a specialist, she was given another depressing diagnosis (cancer, Parkinson's disease), which would later be proven to be incorrect. To forget her gloom, she painted even more, since her hobby always provided her a positive, relaxing outlet. However, it was eventually determined that the paint she used was slowly paralyzing her. Tests confirmed that Barb had n-hexane poisoning. N-hexane is known to cause permanent nerve damage if inhaled frequently. To make matters worse, the rest of her family also had been poisoned. Although not affected to the same degree as Barb, the entire family found it necessary to go through the detox program.

In addition, "fouling the nest" is not just limited to the "nest." My sister told me of a friend of hers who, along with her husband, owned a small pesticide business. One day, my sister sadly watched her friend drive up in none other than the family pest control truck. My sister became even more distraught when she noted that her friend's little two-year-old was happily sitting right next to her mother. Undeniably, both Mom and daughter were being exposed to lingering pesticide vapors as they innocently used the truck for everyday transportation.

Art Supplies and Children

Adult art supplies can cause respiratory and digestive tract problems, skin irritation, organ damage, neurological effects, and cancer. Unfortunately, many children often use or are exposed to adult art supplies. This is of significant concern since children are more at risk from exposures to toxic art products than adults for several reasons.

First, toxic chemicals can enter the bodies of children more easily because they have a faster respiratory rate and thinner skin than adults. Another reason is that children are more likely to misuse products (e.g., taste them, inhale them, throw them, smear them on each other).

Not too long ago, my daughter's play group painted rocks to give as Father's Day gifts. The initial stages of the project seemed quite harmless as the children happily sat outside painting their rocks with watercolors. But then the Mom in charge of the project approached me with a spray can of shellac in her hand. Since she was aware of my chemical sensitivities, she asked if I wanted to forgo spraying my daughter's rock. She was thinking that I would not want the smell on the rock, but I was more immediately concerned that she was going to start spraying all the rocks while our kids were right there. I quickly gathered my own children (and their non-shiny rocks), and put them in the car. Unfortunately, she did not share my concern and began to spray the other children's rocks. As I noted the direction the wind was blowing, the aerosol can she was using, and how close all the other children were to her as she sprayed, I suddenly had this urge to collect *all* the children and put them in my car. I am positive that the shellac she was using was not a children's art product. More than likely, its label carried warnings against inhalation, ingestion, or dermal exposure. Moreover, these children were being exposed to whatever toxic chemicals were in the product just so their rocks could be shiny.

Adult art products are also commonly used in schools. Recently, a survey in New York revealed that schools routinely order rubber cement containing n-hexane (linked to peripheral nerve damage) and permanent markers containing toluene (associated with abnormal liver development) for high school art departments as well as for *elementary schools*. Additionally, acrylic paints containing cadmium (associated with increased lung and prostate cancer) and chromium pigments (known to cause respiratory cancer) were also found in New York school supply inventories. Both cadmium and chromium were proved to be mutagenic in laboratory screening tests.

The Consumer Product Safety Commission (CPSC) has decided that the educational value of art products outweighs their risks. (Under The Consumer Product Safety Act of 1972, the CPSC has the authority to regulate the safety and labeling of art products.) Art materials are exempt from the statute that bans children's products containing hazardous substances. Instead, the Commission has stipulated that some art products must carry warning labels and use instructions, *but it does not require that the products be safe*. Warning labels only need to appear on art products that have been proven hazardous as a result of mortality testing in animals. Mortality testing determines the dose required to kill half a population of laboratory animals within fourteen days. However, the testing does not reveal any information about genetic or organ damage that may result from exposures to lower doses over a longer period of time.

In addition, art supplies designed specifically for children also pose problems, because these too can contain toxic materials. In response to a growing concern over the safety of children's art materials, it is now possible to find products that have either a CP (Certified Product) or AP (Approved Product) seal. Both seals indicate that a product "contains no materials in sufficient quantities to be toxic or injurious to the human body even if ingested."

My sister works in a school district which now only allows "certified" products to be purchased. However, this certification may create a false sense of security, because the approval does not come from an independent government agency overseeing the safety of art products. Rather, the Art & Craft Materials Institute, which is comprised of numerous art supply manufacturers, has created a division that grants CP and AP seals.

There are several problems with this *voluntary* system of regulation. First of all, the three toxicologists making the decisions are employed by the Institute. Secondly, the assessment of safety is strictly based on literature review; the toxicologists do not screen products for chronic health effects that may not be indicated in current literature. Last of all, consumers are expected to accept a CP or AP seal at face value without knowing *all* of the ingredients that are in an art product.

SOLUTIONS AND ALTERNATIVES

REDUCING EXPOSURES TO TERATOGENS AND MUTAGENS

As simple as it sounds, implementing the suggestions in chapters 2, 3, and 4 to reduce exposures to daily chemicals at home will automatically reduce your family's exposures to teratogens and mutagens. However, since so many exposures to toxins occur at work, the following steps can be taken to reduce exposures there.

First, employees are encouraged to gather accurate information about both the type and degree of exposures associated with their job (see the Workplace Questionnaire, Appendix 6, and the Listing of Chemicals Under Study for Reproductive Hazards, Appendix 7). Using this information, employees can then conclude whether or not their jobs pose significant risks. The compiled data can be referred to when voicing concerns to employers and/or when sharing information with other employees. The more employees expressing concerns, the more likely it is management will listen.

According to the OSHA Act of 1970, employers are obligated to "furnish to each of [their] employees employment and a place of employment which are free from recognized hazards that are causing or likely to cause death or serious physical harm." (29 U.S.C. 654 (a)(1). With knowledge of this law, employees can prompt management to rectify any existing work related health hazards. To help employees do this, Jean Stellman, Ph.D., and Susan Daum, M.D., wrote *Work is Dangerous to Your Health*. The book explains how to build a case, collect data, and so forth.

Also, employees can contact the local media, who will often do a story and continue an investigation of their own. Employees can also write state and federal legislators and/or channel grievances through a union (if present). At the very least, employees can take *outdoor* breaks whenever possible.

Ultimately, each individual needs to assess if the income one receives from his or her job outweighs the known health risks. If the risks appear to be great with no sight of change in the immediate future, people need to become creative and determined and find other employment. I believe that the best job and all the money in the world could not even begin to compensate for having a baby born with birth defects.

REDUCING BREAST MILK CONTAMINATION

Many studies have shown a direct correlation between what a woman eats and the amount of residues in her breast milk. For example, in 1976, the EPA analyzed the breast milk of vegetarian women. The study revealed that the levels of pesticide residues in their milk were significantly less than those found in the average non-vegetarian woman's milk. Similar results were found in a study published by the *New England Journal of Medicine*. This study showed the breast milk of vegetarian mothers to contain only 1 or 2 percent of the pesticide contamination found in the milk of non-vegetarian mothers.

Therefore, eliminating non-organic dairy products, meat, poultry, and foods high in fat might significantly reduce the possiblity of breast milk contamination. In addition, women should avoid using pesticides and herbicides and avoid quick weight loss diets during pregnancy and lactation (since dieting mobilizes fat stores causing contaminants to be released into the bloodstream).

While I concur that the facts about breast milk contamination are very disturbing, hopefully, mothers will not become discouraged from breast-feeding. The nutritional, immunological, and psychological benefits of breast-feeding still outweigh any known risks associated with toxic residues in breast milk—especially since baby formulas are also contaminated. Instead, I hope that mothers and mothers-to-be use this knowledge to become motivated to eliminate their exposures to toxins. By doing so, they can feel confident that their nursing infants, who are at the top of the food chain, are receiving mother's milk as it was intended to be.

ALTERNATIVE BABY PRODUCTS

Cloth Diapers

Before I began researching alternative baby care products, I secretly breathed a sigh of relief that my girls are out of diapers so I, personally, would not have to worry about washing a pile of *dirty cloth diapers* (most likely the least toxic alternative to plastic diapers). But now I feel cheated. Not only are cloth diapers safer, but some very smart people have made cloth diapering quite simple too.

The Nikky diaper cover is one popular alternative to using disposable diapers. It is made from breathable natural fibers (cotton and wool) that allow fresh air in to keep a baby's bottom dry without causing a rash. Triple-stitched for strength and double-layered for durability, these diaper covers have no rough edges to chafe or pinch. Each diaper cover has adjustable Velcro closures, so no pins are required.

The Nikky is as easy to use as a disposable diaper. All you do is lay a cloth diaper in the Nikky, inside the waist and leg bands. Then you put the Nikky under your baby, just as you would any diaper, and bring the front panel forward. The sides are tucked in around the baby for a snug fit. Finish up by fastening everything with the Velcro tabs. The entire process takes approximately ten seconds to complete.

A clean Nikky is needed after about three or four changes; therefore, a minimum of three Nikky covers are recommended (since some will be in use, in the wash, and so forth). To clean the covers, machine wash in warm water with a mild soap or detergent that does not contain bleach, borax, softeners, enzymes, or other additives. (Hopefully parents have already replaced toxic laundry detergents with nontoxic ones.) The cotton Nikky covers can be machine dried, while the wool covers should be dried on a line.

Similar to the Nikky is the Bumpkin, which is advertised as an all-in-one washable diaper. The Bumpkin is an oxygen-bleached, dioxin-free cotton diaper joined to a waterproof outer shell made of 100 percent nylon. Only 100 percent cotton flannel touches the baby, while six layers of cotton padding absorb the wetness. The Nikky and the Bumpkin are just two of the many kinds of cloth diapers available today.

I have to admit that the thought of having to clean *any* cloth diapers still does not sound very appealing to me. However, even in the cleaning department, companies have become innovative. For example, two companies, Biobottoms and Baby Bunz & Company, sell the "Diaper Duck"—a nifty tool that wrings out soiled diapers while keeping your hands dry.

I also discovered that using cloth diapers from a diaper service was approximately 500 dollars CHEAPER than buying disposable diapers. If diaper services are not listed in your phone book, a toll-free diaper service information line can help you locate a service near your home (see Appendix 2 for the number).

However, there still may be those occasions when a disposable diaper is needed. The Dovetail, which is free of perfumes, chemicals, plastics, and super-absorbent gels, presently appears to be the best solution. The Dovetail is made from wood pulp, and it biodegrades in one month instead of approximately 500 years, which is how long it takes a regular plastic disposable diaper to break down. Like cloth diapers, the Dovetail is simply placed inside a diaper cover.

Some companies offering alternatives to disposable diapers include: Baby Bunz & Company, Biobottoms, Family Clubhouse, Motherwear, Seventh Generation, and Natural Lifestyle Supplies (see Appendix 2 for addresses). Likewise, these companies and others offer additional nontoxic baby care products.

For example, to clean a baby's bottom, Seventh Generation offers dioxin-free, alcohol-free, and scent-free baby wipes made from lanolin. As another alternative to baby wipes, Motherwear offers small, 100-percent cotton washcloths. Motherwear also offers a simple herbal salve that is effective against diaper rash and chafing and an unscented, unpetroleum jelly, called Vegelatum, made completely from plant derivatives.

Autumn Harp has its own unpetroleum jelly, along with talc-free baby powder, and an extra-mild baby shampoo. Natural Lifestyle Supplies also offers a line of nontoxic baby care products, including baby shampoos, baby soap, baby oil, baby cream, and a talc-free baby powder. (See Appendix 2 for addresses.)

These products and companies only begin to show the variety of nontoxic alternatives available to concerned parents. I became very excited when I learned how many products and companies were already committed to producing nontoxic baby products. (In fact, I have already planned every nontoxic baby item for my poor sister who has only just recently become engaged.) I think the fact that parents can choose from a variety of nontoxic products makes the decision to use nontoxic products even more appealing. I hope all parents decide to surround their baby with plenty of love *and* nontoxic baby care products.

Nontoxic Toys

When my first daughter was born, one of my friends gave her a hand carved, wooden rattle. Although I remember admiring its beautiful craftsmanship, at the time I did not appreciate how wonderful a gift it truly was.

With my present knowledge of chemicals, I now find myself cringing when I watch babies sucking on plastic rattles or any other toys made from toxic materials. Since babies put almost everything into their mouths, I think it is very important to note what materials baby toys are made of. I now would much rather have my baby put a wooden rattle or toy in his or her mouth instead of a plastic one.

In researching for this book, I sent away for many catalogs from companies that make toys from natural materials, such as wood and cotton (see Appendix 2 for names and addresses). Looking at the catalogs made me somewhat nostalgic, because the toys reminded me of the quality items that used to be found in toy stores long before plastic came along. For those who may doubt the appeal of these toys to children, my two young girls were just as impressed with the toys in catalog as I was ("Oooh—can we have that? How about that?"). While these toys are generally more expensive, they will probably last longer since they are made of quality materials.

However, since the majority of the toys on the market today are not made of natural materials, it is probably unrealistic to expect that a synthetic toy will never enter your home. For example, Barbie and her gang are more popular today than ever—and I've yet to come across a Barbie made out of natural materials.

Rather than ban the sacred Barbie from our home, we have reached a compromise that suits the whole family. Even my daughters cannot deny how much a new Barbie "smells." Our solution is that our new Barbies become great campers—all of them must first sleep outside to outgas. In fact, when a friend gave my youngest daughter a big plastic Barbie case for her birthday, it was Kiley who said, in reference to the smell of the outgassing chemicals and not the present, "It stinks—better put it outside." After the initial outgassing has decreased, and Barbie is brought inside, Barbie (like all other synthetic toys) is kept in a room other than our daughters' bedroom.

With my new knowledge of chemicals, I am also now somewhat skeptical when I see the word "nontoxic" printed on a toy package. A distressing, recurring theme of this book is the fact that information printed on a product label (such as "natural" or "biodegradable") may not always be accurate. My new guideline is to look further to see if any "precautions" are also listed (even though I know this guideline is not foolproof either). For example, my family and I were in a small souvenir shop when my children spotted a package of "magic" dinosaurs. The package explained that the little pellets in the package turned into dinosaurs when immersed in water. The word NONTOXIC was plastered all over the package in bold print. But in the fine, small print, parents were warned that the pellets should not be swallowed.

I do not know if this product was harmful or not. However, the "warning" was enough to deter me. While some may find my decision overly protective, I honestly do not believe that my children can be called underprivileged because a stegosaurus will not be materializing in their bath.

The Nontoxic Nursery

All of the alternatives discussed in chapter 3 for reducing toxins in the home are applicable to creating a safe baby's room. A nontoxic nursery would have: walls painted with nontoxic paint; tile, natural linoleum, or hardwood flooring laid with nontoxic glues; all pressed wood furniture sealed with a nontoxic sealant; a futon crib mattress made out of organically grown cotton; bedding made out of 100-percent cotton; nontoxic baby care products; and toys made from natural materials (other toys are kept in another room). Likewise, the room would be cleaned with nontoxic cleaners (see Appendix 2) and, in all cases, any kind of pest control used in or around the room would be nontoxic. (Around the room includes the outdoors as well. For example, if parents spray the bushes outside the baby's room and open the window the next day, the baby will inhale the pesticides.)

I know we tend to think that everything for our baby should be fresh and new. But in general, the words OLD and HANDED-DOWN should be the key words when creating a nontoxic nursery. Most baby items, especially furniture, do not get worn out since your baby only uses them for a short period of time. Therefore, not only is it healthier for your baby to use furniture and other baby items that are not brand new, but it is more practical and economical.

At the very least, parents should try to finish decorating the nursery many months prior to the birth of their child. If parents are still determined to lay new carpet, it should be installed seven or eight months before the baby is born. This way, the room can be aired out repeatedly before the baby is brought home, and the baby will not be exposed to the initial outgassing vapors, which are the most harmful. (However, keep in mind that carpet, paint, furniture, etc., will continue to outgas even after the initial strong vapors have disappeared.)

To help parents evaluate the amount of toxins in a nursery, I have created the Baby Room Questionnaire (Appendix 8). If upon completion of this sheet, parents are satisfied that they have decorated the nursery with a minimal amount of chemical products, then they will not need to make changes. But, if upon completion it becomes obvious that their baby is going to be exposed to countless chemicals from the minute he or she arrives home, perhaps some modifications can be made.

I promise, your baby will thank you for it. And, if you are still bothered that your baby's nursery did not turn out as you had once envisioned, be reassured that it is a rare, rare child that can even recall what his or her nursery looked like (can you?).

CREATING A NONTOXIC NEST

The first step for keeping contaminants out of the "nest" is to understand what chemicals are harmful and how they may be entering the home.

As a general rule, persons who work with chemicals should remove all work clothing (including shoes) as well as work tools before entering their homes. Ideally, workplaces should have locker rooms where employees can shower and change, thus eliminating the need for employees to wear their work clothes home. If such a facility is not available, workers can remove and store their clothes and tools in their garage at home. Persons who come in contact with chemicals at their job should always shower after work.

Keep in mind that the nest is not only fouled by contaminants brought home from work. If your garage is attached to your house and it has not been sealed, it can also be fouling the nest. Toxic vapors from whatever is stored in the garage, such as pesticides, paint, and gasoline, can easily enter and contaminate your home.

Most people are already very protective of their homes. Therefore, it is my hope that people will want to make a conscious effort to keep their home/nest clean and uncontaminated. While we may not always be able to do this in work environments or other places in the community, we *can* successfully create a loving, NONTOXIC home environment for our children.

Art Without Toxic Exposures

According to the Natural Resources Defense Council, which puts out a comprehensive report called "Children's Art Hazards" by Lauren Jacobson, the following art materials are considered hazardous for children under the age of twelve and should not be used by them at any time: acrylics, alkyd paints, oil paints, phosphorescent paints, India ink, airplane glue, epoxy glue, instant glue, rubber cement, spray adhesives, varnish and wood stains, artists pastels, permanent marking pens, household and direct dyes, cold water fiber reactive dyes, professional ceramic glazes, metal enameling glaze powders, and solvents (e.g., turpentine, acetone, hexane).

The Council has recommended that the following products be used with caution, meaning that the amount of the product used and the number of times it is used should be monitored: tempura or poster paints, wheat paste, white or library paste, water-based marking pens, vegetable and natural plant dyes (make sure that the dye is made from a non-poisonous plant), and instant paper mache (use only ground cellulose variety).

Based on available ingredient information, the following materials are considered safe: finger paints, water colors, white glue, chalk, crayons, school (dustless) pastels, pencils, and modeling clay (or playdough).

Many safe (or at least safer) alternatives can be substituted for hazardous products. For example, use talc-free, premixed clay instead of clay in the dry form; use water-based paints instead of ceramic glazes and copper enamels; use vegetable, plant, or food dyes instead of commercial dyes; use liquid or pre-mixed paints rather than powdered tempera colors; and use water-based products rather than turpentine, shellac, or rubber cement. You can also substitute water-based paints for aerosol spray paints; white glue or wheat paste for epoxy or airplane glue; water-based markers for permanent, scented felt tip markers; and medical plaster for casting plaster.

The Council advises that children should avoid using all professional art supplies, any product with a label carrying special use instructions or first-aid warnings, and any products with artificial fruit or food scents. (Scented products may attract children to taste or eat them.)

In addition, to minimize the risk of children inhaling toxic vapors from art products, parents and teachers should wipe or wet mop instead of sweeping when cleaning up after art projects. Likewise, children should always wash their hands after working on projects to prevent skin irritation, which may result from contact with certain art supplies.

Current federal legislation could be greatly improved to assist parents and teachers in protecting children from exposures to hazardous art products. Proposed legislation changes which are supported by the Natural Defense Resource Council include: requiring that all ingredients that are present at a level of 0.1 percent or more in an art product be listed on the label, requiring toxicity screening tests for art products, and requiring that all chronic and acute health hazards be listed on the product label.

Remember—creativity and imagination are probably an artist's most viable tools—and both are unquestionably nontoxic. Certainly, budding young artists can be encouraged without exposing them to hazardous art materials. After all, we would like to first ensure that these promising, creative children *do* grow up.

IN THE FUTURE

I have a friend who, although she was interested in hearing about the problems with traditional products, never specifically inquired about any of the nontoxic alternatives until her first child was born just a month ago. Now, suddenly, as my friend holds this precious new life in her arms, she has a list of questions for me, and she wants the names of nontoxic products.

I am glad. If some people have difficulty in becoming motivated to make nontoxic changes for themselves, then I am hoping that the incredible joy a parent experiences when an infant falls asleep on his or her shoulder or smiles for the first time or takes his or her first step will trigger a commitment to surround that child with the best, nontoxic environment possible.

I admit that when reviewing the information about chemicals and babies, it suddenly seems as if sterilized bottles and bumper pads are just not enough to ensure our children's health and safety. Fortunately, various organizations, resources, and manufacturers have known this for quite a while. They provide numerous nontoxic alternatives for parents (see Appendix 2, "Specifically for Children").

Legislation is also beginning to address the impact exposures to certain chemicals can have on reproductive function. In fact, it is not uncommon (though certainly still not the norm) to see signs posted on buildings warning expectant mothers that teratogenic chemicals are present.

Presently, the responsibility for reducing their children's exposures to toxins falls primarily on parents. That is no small responsibility. Even before I became aware of the potential impact chemicals can have on children, I had always thought that motherhood was a tremendous responsibility. But I had never really thought about my responsibility extending beyond my own children. It was not until I began reading and writing about mutagens that I finally internalized that some of my daily decisions could affect *the next several generations of my family.*

With my new knowledge of mutagens, I now find it impossible to concur with parents who point to their family's present good health as proof that the chemicals in their lives are having no adverse effect on them. I wonder if these parents will feel the same if sometime in the future they discover that their children are sterile—or find themselves grandparents to grandchildren with birth defects. But I hope this never happens. Instead, I hope that individuals will acknowledge that there is enough documented information about chemicals and reproductive function to start making some changes right now.

CHECKLIST FOR SUGGESTED CHANGES AND COMMITMENTS

- ☐ Avoid, as much as possible, exposures to any chemicals (including daily household cleaners, etc.) while pregnant or nursing.
- ☐ When planning a family, complete the Work Survey (Appendix 7) to evaluate whether or not either spouses' work environment exposes him or her to toxic chemicals.
- ☐ If the results of the Work Survey warrant justifiable concern, organize a group to urge employers to provide a safe work environment (in accordance with the OSHA Act of 1970).
- ☐ If your employer refuses to modify an unsafe work environment, seriously consider finding another job or seek a position within the same company that may not be as hazardous.
- ☐ In order to reduce breast milk contamination, nursing mothers should reduce or eliminate meat, pork, poultry, and dairy products from their diets. (This also applies to women who are not breast-feeding but who are planning to start a family, since a mother's past exposures can contaminate breast milk also.)

☐ When breast-feeding, avoid any quick weight loss diets since rapid weight loss can increase breast milk contamination.

☐ Buy children's clothing made from natural fibers (see Appendix 2).

☐ Purchase toys made from natural materials (see Appendix 2).

☐ Make sure all new toys (especially those with strong plastic smells) out-gas outside.

☐ Find a place (other than the child's room) to store synthetic toys.

☐ Use only nontoxic cleaners in the baby's room (see Appendix 2).

☐ Avoid using any kind of pesticides in or around the baby's room.

☐ Use nontoxic baby care products (see Appendix 2).

☐ Use cloth diapers.

☐ Purchase a crib mattress that has been made with 100 percent, organically grown cotton or untreated wool (see Appendix 2).

☐ Use a nontoxic sealant to seal any pressed wood furniture in the baby's room (see Appendix 2).

☐ Using nontoxic glue, lay alternative flooring (natural linoleum, hardwood floors, or tile) in the baby's room (see Appendix 2).

☐ If using any toxic materials to decorate the baby's room, do so at least six or seven months prior to the birth of the baby. During this time, the room should be well-ventilated and aired out.

☐ Encourage children to wash their hands after working with art supplies.

☐ Clean up art projects by wiping or wet mopping rather than sweeping.

☐ Avoid using the following art products around children: aerosol art products or airbrush techniques, solvents, or glazes.

☐ Avoid purchasing art products that have artificial fruit or food scents.

☐ Do not allow children to use or be around adult professional art materials.

☐ Work with your child's school district to implement a policy for using only safe art materials in classrooms.

☐ Support legislation changes that would require the following: that all elementary and secondary school teachers pass a course on the potential hazards of art supplies; more accurate labeling of ingredients in art supplies; toxicity screening tests for art supplies; identification of all chronic and acute health hazards associated with an art product.

Quiz 6—A Pretest on Allergic Children

1. According to Dr. Marshall Mandall, a child experiencing reoccurring fatigue along with a stuffy nose and/or mental confusion/depression may _____.

    A) have a mold and/or yeast sensitivity

    B) have chronic sinusitis

    C) need psychological counseling

2. When a child develops an allergic condition, his or her detoxification system _____.

    A) can be improved by taking antihistamine drugs

    B) has most likely become impaired

3. The "spreading phenomenon" (in regards to an allergic condition) refers to the fact that _____.

    A) allergic conditions may be contagious

    B) individuals who initially become sensitized to a few chemicals may start reacting to other chemicals that have never previously bothered them

    C) more and more doctors are beginning to understand the cause and effect relationship between chemicals and ill-health

4. _____ is now the leading reason children are hospitalized in the United States. [1]

    A) Diabetes

    B) Asthma

    C) Measles

5. Provocation/neutralization methods of allergy testing _____.

    A) do not work with children under the age of twelve

    B) can enable a physician to reproduce symptoms with one dilution of an extract and eliminate them with another

6. Children with chemical sensitivities often _____.

    A) complain of odors others do not notice

    B) cannot smell odors that most people can

7. The _____ is usually the primary target organ when a person's detoxification system becomes impaired.[2]

    A) heart

    B) brain

    C) gall bladder

8. According to a report in the *Journal of the American Medical Association*, the use of Ritalin and other drugs to treat hyperactivity has doubled every _____.[3]

        A) ten to fifteen years
        B) twenty to thirty years
        C) four to seven years

Answers to Allergic Children Quiz

1. A Although molds and yeast are very different, they are part of the same fungi family. Therefore, a person who is sensitive to one may be sensitive to the other. Yeast can be found in breads, crackers, pretzels, pastries, and milk fortified with vitamins from yeast. In addition, vinegars and all fruit juices contain yeast forming substances. Foods that contain mold include mushrooms, cheeses of all kinds, and dried herbs. In the home, mold can commonly be found near tubs and sinks; in soil; in carpets; inside mattresses, stuffed furniture, or air conditioners; or in any area which has been damaged by water (e.g., ceilings, basements).

2. B Antihistamine drugs may help alleviate symptoms, but they will do nothing to improve a weakened detoxification system. In contrast, comprehensive allergy care under a skilled clinical ecologist will strengthen the detoxification system and help alleviate symptoms. When a child becomes "overloaded" with chemical exposures, his or her detoxification system may become dysfunctional causing a backlog of toxic chemicals to build up in the body. Treating the *entire* detoxification system, as opposed to just treating visible symptoms, will be the most effective way of reducing and/or eliminating the allergic condition.

3. B Typically, individuals develop *multiple* sensitivities to foods and/ or chemicals. Therefore, health may not improve until all environmental triggers have been identified.

4. B In 1988, one out of every five children with asthma was hospitalized. Despite modern medicine's attempts to treat asthma, the asthma death rate *rose 30 percent* between 1983 and 1987 in the United States. Moreover, since 1970, the number of people estimated to have asthma has doubled from six million to twelve million. A recent study published in the *New England Journal of Medicine* concludes that virtually all asthma attacks are triggered by allergies.

5. B This form of allergy testing is practiced by clinical ecologists. A patient, who can even be a very small child, is given a small extract of a suspected allergen. Reactions are then noted. Typically, a whole range of symptoms occurs almost immediately if the patient is sensitive to the allergen. Next, a "neutralizing" dose of the same allergen is given that almost immediately makes the symptoms disappear.

6. A   An unusual sensitivity to odors can be an excellent clue that a person suffers from chemical sensitivities.

7. B   The brain is usually the target organ because so many of the chemicals which enter the body's bloodstream are lipid soluble, and lipids are abundant in the brain and nervous system.

8. C   The prognosis of hyperactive children who are only treated with medication is not encouraging. In fact, boys who take medication for hyperactivity are considered to be at high risk for having problems at school and with the law. Likewise, if a child is hyperactive because he or she has a dysfunctional detoxification system, medicating the child will only aggravate the problem in the long run. In contrast, making dietary changes, reducing chemical exposures, and giving nutritional supplements in combination with psychological support has proven to bring about remarkable changes in some hyperactive children.

CHAPTER SIX

Today's "Allergic" Children

While I was making other changes in my life to improve my health, I had food allergy testing done since I was certain that some foods had also affected me. I had often experienced tiredness, a distended abdomen and gas after eating. Nothing too serious, but enough to be bothersome.

The type of food testing that my doctor used is called provocation-neutralization. It is very different from the standard allergy scratch test. In the provocation-neutralization test, a minute extract of a specific allergen is either placed under the tongue or injected under the skin. Afterwards, the patient is monitored to see if the antigen causes any physical or behavioral reactions. In order to prevent any pre-disposed biases towards the food (or chemical substance) being tested, the patient is not told what food or substance is being injected. If the patient does react to the antigen, a "neutralizing" dose of the same extract is administered until the symptoms subside.

Eager to discover which foods were having an adverse affect on me, I entered the allergy room of the doctor's office in a very good mood and with lots of energy. I even smiled sweetly as the nurse injected me with the first extract.

I was then told to wait ten minutes. I experienced no itching or swelling at the injection site, only a slight redness. The nurse then injected me again with a little higher dose of the "mystery" food.

I confidently returned to my seat, convinced that the nurse was, of course, starting out with foods that I had said didn't cause reactions in me. So, I was quite surprised when seconds later I suddenly became weak. I then experienced an avalanche of other symptoms. Immediately, my throat swelled and my ears and nose became congested.

But then came the biggest surprise: I began to feel extremely depressed. Sitting in a room full of strangers, I desperately, but unsuccessfully, tried to

191

hide the tears that were streaming down my cheeks. Not only was the aller-gen triggering physical reactions, but it was triggering behavioral reactions as well!

It seemed like the ten-minute waiting period would never end. As the time dragged on, I convinced myself that all these symptoms could not pos-sibly have been caused by the injection. I did not believe that a food could cause such symptoms. Instead, I thought I must have been reacting to some other kind of toxin.

When the ten minutes were up, the nurse gave me my first trial dose of antigen. But the antigen made no difference; I continued to suffer from the symptoms. By now, I had become completely convinced that what was hap-pening to me had nothing to do with food. My depression was slowly turn-ing into illogical anger. (I was thinking the most unpleasant thoughts about the poor nurse.) I could not even begin to figure out how I was going to get home in that condition.

Ten minutes later, I received another dose of antigen. This time, miracu-lously, the antigen worked, and my storm subsided. All of my symptoms, in-cluding the depression, began to disappear. I was astonished.

I looked at the nurse and asked incredulously, "Tell me, what *was* the food?"

"Chicken," she responded.

I shook my head in disbelief. I had never thought I was sensitive to chicken. But then I remembered back several weeks to the Fourth of July. The day had been a confusing setback for me. I had felt well in the morning as we watched the city's parade, and later when we picnicked at the beach. But by late afternoon, I was experiencing symptoms like those I had had in the doctor's office. Only because it was a holiday did I remember what I had eaten for lunch that day—chicken.

I had known that reactions to foods can occur immediately after eating the food or as long as twenty-four hours later. But never once did I realize the intensity of the symptoms that a *food sensitivity* could cause. Previously, I had thought I only experienced severe reactions to *chemical exposures*. More and more, the concept of an allergy was expanding to have new mean-ing for me.

Later, I began to realize that many allergies are symptoms of a person's having an impaired detox system. I discovered that when the body's detoxi-fication system is strengthened and repaired many of these allergies disap-pear.

Although the word allergy has been around since 1906, not all doctors today agree on what can cause allergies. Most doctors accept that individuals can be allergic to molds, pollens, and dust and have symptoms such as hay fever, sinus infections, and asthma. But many doctors do not accept the premise that *anything* in the environment can trigger almost any kind of allergic reaction, depending on the individual and the current state of his or her detoxification system.

This chapter will explore how allergic reactions and a malfunctioning detoxification system can cause a variety of physical symptoms (e.g., ear infections, muscle aches, bed-wetting) and negative behaviors (e.g., temper tantrums, biting, hyperactivity). I hope that the information in this chapter will help parents to determine whether or not their child has an impaired detox system and, if so, help them to become motivated to improve their child's health.

While I have named this chapter "Today's Allergic Child," I am hoping that after reading this information parents will understand that treating a child's allergies goes far beyond treating immediate allergic symptoms. I am hoping that parents will come to view allergies as a *symptom* of an impaired detoxification system.

I have a great desire to share what I have learned about the human detoxification system primarily because I think the information applies to everyone. Learning about the detoxification system can help us understand how many of the chemicals I have thus discussed may be having a negative impact on you and your family—even if no symptoms are present right now. An understanding of the body's detoxification system can help explain how someone can appear to be well one day and then suddenly start to have unexplainable symptoms almost overnight. This understanding can also explain how the chemicals in our lives can and do affect behavior, mood, concentration, and overall academic performance.

THE PROBLEMS

OVERLOADED DETOXIFICATION SYSTEMS

I was first prompted to learn about the body's detoxification system after I discovered that many of the patients at the detox clinic had been there before. These patients told me that they *had* felt better after detoxing the first time, but that when they resumed their ordinary lifestyles they filled up with chemicals again. As a result, they returned to the clinic whenever their symptoms once again became too unbearable.

The thought of ever having to return to the detox clinic greatly concerned me. I had already concluded that the clinic was one of the most stressful and depressing places imaginable. Furthermore, I started thinking that some of the patients were using the detox clinic in the same way some people use over-the-counter or prescription drugs—as a temporary solution for alleviating a symptom. I concluded that these patients and I were not addressing the real source of our problem—*why* we had filled up with toxins in the first place.

My concerns and questions motivated me to learn about the body's detoxification system. I wanted to fully understand how I had become so ill from exposures to everyday chemicals and why others did not appear to be affected. After acquiring this invaluable information, I suddenly knew what I needed to do to regain my health. To truly get better, I discovered that I had to do more than just detox the chemicals stored in my body. I also needed to repair my malfunctioning detoxification system, which, most likely, had made me so vulnerable to the chemicals in the first place.

Dr. Sherry Rogers, a well-known doctor who not only treats patients with impaired detoxification systems but teaches the advanced physicians course on this subject, explains the detoxification system in detail in her latest book, *Tired or Toxic?* While I cannot begin to address the subject in the thorough, comprehensive manner that she does, I will attempt to summarize the major points.

However, I want to preface the following explanation of the body's detox system by sharing the dilemma I faced when preparing my thoughts. I recognize that there are some people, such as my husband, who will always want precise, technical explanations, and will, therefore, welcome and appreciate specific references and scientific terminology. Yet, I also recognize that there are others who simply become intimidated and/or bored by such explanations. I have tried to keep both persons in mind when writing about the detoxification system. In order to provide the reader with some understanding of how this system can fail, I have focused primarily on the different ways a detoxification system can become impaired. But, I have chosen not to include detailed explanations of the cellular biochemistry of the detoxification process, because I fear that those who do not need such information will get lost (or bored). For those of you seeking a more thorough explanation, please refer to Rogers' *Tired or Toxic?*

The primary function of the detoxification system is to keep the body clean and healthy. When it is functioning properly, even toxic chemicals are broken down and excreted. However, since we are exposed to so many chemicals, this system can often become overloaded or impaired, resulting in numerous symptoms or chronic illness.

To understand the body's detox system and how it can become impaired, it is first important to realize that everything we breathe (whether we smell it or not), eat, or absorb through our skin enters our bloodstream. When a chemical enters our blood, one of three things happens. First (and ideally), the body can excrete the chemical. If the body cannot (for reasons I will explain shortly), the body may then store the chemical in fat or vital body tissues until the body is able to excrete it at a later time (recall that breast-feeding is such an opportunity). Lastly, the body may turn the chemical into something even more toxic, which increases the probability of permanent damage to the detoxification system and/or body organs.

Detoxification occurs in two phases. In Phase I of the detoxification process, the body breaks down the chemical at the cellular level to make the chemical less toxic and sends it to the kidneys to be excreted. During Phase I, the body first breaks down some chemicals into an alcohol. Next, the alcohol is metabolized into an aldehyde, the aldehyde is transformed into an acid, and the acid is excreted through the urine.

There are several enzyme-related factors that affect this phase of detoxification. Very specific enzymes are needed to break down different chemicals into alcohol. However, many of the enzymes that are necessary for this process to occur depend on specific vitamins and minerals in order to function. In some cases, without the presence of a particular nutrient, the enzyme is ineffective. For example, the mineral zinc is needed to transform alcohol into aldehyde, and the mineral molybdenum is needed to transform aldehyde into acid. If a person is deficient in these minerals, the detoxification process fails. The body may make choral hydrate instead of aldehyde. Choral hydrate affects brain function, making a person feel "drunk."

It is also possible that both the enzymes and nutrients are present, but that they cannot detox a chemical because they are tied up trying to detox other chemicals. This happens when the body is overburdened with chemicals (e.g., from simultaneous exposure to new carpet, paint, pesticides, and so forth). Or, it may be that an individual just does not possess the necessary enzyme. Last of all, it is possible that past chemical exposures have destroyed the enzyme necessary for detoxing a particular chemical (how this happens will be explained shortly).

Chemicals that are not excreted to the kidneys during Phase I, pass on to Phase II of the detoxification process. During Phase II, a large protein or amino acid hooks on to the chemical (from Phase I). The chemical can then easily be excreted through the bile and pass into the stool. This process is dependent upon a chemical compound of three amino acids—glutamine, glycine, and cysteine, a combination referred to as GSH. GSH helps the body detox foreign chemicals, medications, and radiation, and it directly and in-

directly affects many other important body functions (e.g., making new genetic material, enzymes, and hormones).

However, each time a molecule of GSH is attached to a chemical, the
body permanently loses that molecule of GSH. If a person's supply of GSH
becomes depleted by being constantly called upon to help detox in Phase II,
it eventually becomes difficult for a person to even tolerate normal, everyday exposures to chemicals.

If major alcohol and aldehyde detoxification paths become impaired,
the body may then make *epoxides*, highly reactive and unstable chemicals,
from the chemicals not broken down in either phase I or II. Epoxides are
products of a metabolic process and are capable of initiating cancer (by at-
taching to DNA), allergies, environmental illness, immunosuppression,
changes in genetics, and birth defects.

For those (like myself) who are not scientifically-minded, it might be
helpful to envision epoxides as wayward toxic chemicals that roam the
body, creating havoc until they can be detoxed in an alternate pathway.
During this time, these chemicals are capable of causing permanent damage
to the enzymes that are needed for the detoxification system to work as intended.

Also, when normal detox pathways are not functioning optimally,
chemicals in need of a pathway might "crowd" into another pathway, inter-
fering with the detoxification of the chemical already in that pathway.
When this occurs, neither chemical can be easily detoxed. Subsequently, the
detoxification system becomes even further impaired, and a person experiences more symptoms from their chemical exposures. Once the detox system becomes dysfunctional, the damage becomes exponential, and a person
may experience a rapid downward spiral in health.

Even if a person begins to reduce the amount of toxic chemicals he or
she is exposed to, the person's detoxification system may still never function
optimally again because there may have been permanent damage to cells.
Even though I am doing all I can to repair my own detoxification system, I
cannot predict whether or not I will one day be able to tolerate common, everyday chemicals like other people do.

I continue to be fascinated by all this information—especially when I
think about how I have been able to improve my health now that I understand the detoxification process. What is still so utterly amazing to me is
that I became so critically ill (many believe that I had come very close to dying) when I filled my life and body with chemicals and how much stronger
and healthier I have become now that I have begun to reverse the process by
greatly reducing the chemicals in my life and simultaneously repairing my
detoxification system.

My own plan for repairing my impaired detoxification system includes eating a macrobiotic diet (which eliminates my body's need to detox the chemicals found in a traditional diet and provides me with important nutrients necessary to the overall detoxification process), taking additional specific nutrients for those vitamins and minerals that I was so deficient in that even a macrobiotic diet could not supply them (it should be noted that individuals should not take nutrient supplements without the guidance of a doctor trained in this area; many nutrients can be harmful if taken in large doses), reducing as much as possible the chemicals in my home and life, taking two to four saunas a week, and having a weekly massage and occasional acupuncture treatments.

I sometimes find myself comparing this self-healing approach to the traditional approach I followed when I first became sick, the one that led to three surgeries, countless prescriptions, and which, subsequently, just got me sicker and sicker. Of course, I now realize that the anesthesia from the surgeries and the never-ending medications were just more chemicals (on top of all the pesticides and formaldehyde that I was continually exposed to in my home) that my poor body had to detox.

I also now understand why my present plan for improving my health is working—and why, in many ways, it is actually helping me to achieve a level of health I had never experienced prior to becoming ill. It is working because what is wrong with me is not a sinus condition or a pituitary tumor or asthma or Addison's disease (to name just a few of my past diagnoses). What is wrong with me is that I have a dysfunctional detoxification system. That is the real source of all my symptoms. Unfortunately, many other people continue to suffer the adverse effects of a dysfunctional detoxification system without realizing that it is also the source of their symptoms.

The Masking Phenomenon (or Why Some People Think They Are Unaffected by Chemicals)

Many people may find it hard to accept that chemicals are harming them since they currently don't exhibit any symptoms. Most people have been taught to believe that the absence of symptoms is the equivalent of good health. However, most people probably do not realize that it is possible for symptoms of toxic exposures to be *masked*. The *masking phenomenon* is the body's natural ability to adapt to continual toxic exposures. The masking phenomenon occurs when the body starts to increase production of the particular enzyme needed to detox whatever toxin is repeatedly entering the bloodstream.

As enzyme production increases, symptoms that may have originally resulted from the toxic exposure become masked. This explains why people will often admit that a chemical exposure, such as from new carpet or fresh paint, bothered them at first, causing symptoms such as headaches and respiratory problems, but that after a few weeks their symptoms "disappeared." More than likely their original symptoms have not "disappeared" but are merely being masked.

Besides allowing people to falsely believe that exposures to toxic chemicals are not affecting them, the masking phenomenon places tremendous stress on the body. Masking requires a great deal of enzymes and nutrients. When so many enzymes and nutrients have to be devoted to masking, the entire detox system becomes adversely affected. As a result, a person may begin to feel chronically fatigued or experience other symptoms seemingly unrelated to the original symptoms. In addition, there is a limit to how long a person's body can "adapt" to chemical exposures by masking symptoms. At some point, some people's bodies will just break down.

Smoking is a good example of how the masking phenomenon works. When people take their first puffs on a cigarette, they usually cough and gag. That is the body's natural response to inhaling cigarette smoke, the body's natural warning sign that smoking is not healthy. However, if a person continues to smoke, eventually the body will adapt, and its natural response to smoking will be masked. However, just because the coughing and gagging have stopped does not mean that smoking is no longer harming a person.

Just as it is possible to mask symptoms, it is also possible to *unmask* symptoms. When exposure to a certain toxic substance is reduced or eliminated for a specific period of time, the enzyme level stops being elevated. For example, if a smoker stops smoking for a year and then starts again, he or she will probably cough and gag again upon taking that first puff because the body's natural response to smoking has become *unmasked.*

The masking phenomenon does not just apply to chemicals either. Adverse sensitivities to food and drink can also be masked. For example, when I first met my husband, he always needed at least three cups of coffee in the morning to get him going. He was like a zombie without it. Not surprisingly, on the morning he decided to give up coffee he was so lethargic by noon (and in the foulest mood) that I wasn't sure he was going to even be able to make it up the stairs to take a nap. He also claimed that he had the worst headache he had ever had in his entire life. His body's natural response to caffeine was becoming unmasked; he was suffering withdrawal symptoms like an addict.

His second morning without coffee was not much better; the third was only a slight improvement. It was almost a week before he could awaken and feel refreshed without coffee.

Some people seem to be great adapters. They adapt and adapt until one day they discover they have cancer. My father is such an example. For seventy years he was never sick. Then, almost overnight, he was diagnosed with lymphatic cancer. A year after treatment, another malignant tumor was discovered, and eight months later he was diagnosed with cancer of the bladder. (It should be noted that my father has opted for standard cancer treatment, instead of alternative medicine, and has made no lifestyle or diet changes—with the exception of giving up his pipe).

In the case of my father, some might say, "Well, he *is* in his seventies....," implying that when people reach a certain age it is almost inevitable that they will become sick. However, the time period between when exposures to carcinogens occur and a malignancy shows up is considered to be twenty to thirty years. This means that the exposures that triggered my father's cancers occurred when he was forty or fifty, sometime during the 1960s or 1970s, or, in other words, during a time when we know the world had already become inundated with chemicals. My concern is that if it takes twenty to thirty years for cancer to be manifested, children today, who are living in an even more chemically-dependent world than my father did, might right now be surrounded by and masking toxic exposures that will later initiate cancer. However, unlike my father who developed cancer in his seventies, these children will develop cancer in their twenties and thirties. Unfortunately, this is already happening. Sadly, the daughter of friends of our family has just recently died of lung cancer; she was in her thirties. She makes the fourth person *under the age of forty* that I personally know of who has died of cancer.

Does Your Child Have an Impaired Detoxification System?

Considering the possible effects an impaired detoxification system can have, it is important to evaluate whether or not the detoxification system of the average child is functioning optimally. We can start this evaluation by focusing on the average American diet. Since we now know that specific nutrients are needed for Phase I and Phase II of the detoxification process, it is alarming to note how many of these nutrients are missing from the typical American diet. According to Dr. Mildred Seelig, one of the country's leading authorities on magnesium, approximately 80 to 90 percent of the population is notably deficient in this mineral.[4] Nearly 300 enzymes depend on magnesium in order to function.

However, magnesium is hardly the only nutrient missing from the typical American diet. Commercial produce, because it is grown with so many chemicals, has fewer nutrients than organic produce. Commercial produce may have only 25 percent of the total nutrients found in organic produce.

The high level of phosphates found in soda drinks and other processed foods also interferes with the absorption of minerals. Sugar, which seems to be in almost every processed food, also depletes the body of vitamins and minerals. Moreover, vitamin E may be missing from the average American's diet since it is often removed from most grocery store oil and flour during processing. Vitamin E is instrumental to the body's detox system because it helps prevent cell membranes from being destroyed by epoxides.

What is currently happening in Japan may be a very good example of how the traditional American diet might trigger allergies. The traditional diet of Japan consists of rice, fish, tofu, seaweed and fresh vegetables. However, many young people in Japan today are eating a diet that is comparable to the diet eaten by many American youngsters—a diet high in processed foods. A recent study done by Japan's Food Industry Center revealed that not one traditional Japanese dish ranked in the top ten food choices of junior high students.

The effect of this dietary change in Japan has stunned the Education Ministry. The Ministry recently ordered a three-year nationwide survey of the health of *all* school children in Japan. A preliminary study of 2,660 Japanese elementary and high school students revealed an undeniable, steady deterioration in these youngster's health. Specifically, 90.8 percent of them suffer from allergies—compared to 72 percent in 1978. There were also significant increases in the number of children who suffer from skin problems, chronic fatigue, back pain, and diabetes.[5] The increase of allergies and illness among Japanese children now eating an American diet suggests that this diet may impair a child's detoxification system and general health.

Another factor to consider when evaluating the condition of the average person's detoxification system is the increased construction of energy-tight buildings and homes that has occurred since the 1970s. More and more synthetic chemicals are now being used in building materials, carpets, furniture, clothing, and personal care products, which means that individuals who live or work in energy-tight structures (which, by their very nature, have poor ventilation) are forced to inhale increased levels of toxins.

Other factors that can affect the condition of a person's detoxification system include our heavy reliance on pesticides, herbicides, and fungicides to keep homes, schools, and commercial·environments surrounded by green lawns and free of pests; the contamination of the water which we drink and bathe in; and the pollution of the air we breathe by toxic chemicals. Moreover, of the 48,000 chemicals listed by the EPA, there are virtually no studies on the toxic human effect for almost 80 percent of them.[6] And, as if that were not enough, approximately one thousand new synthetic chemical compounds are introduced each year.

No doubt about it, we live in a very chemical world. From the minute they are born and for the rest of their lives, our children are forced to detox toxic chemicals. Considering the many factors that can easily affect the effectiveness of the detoxification system and how many chemicals are now so intertwined with our lives, I find it impossible to conclude that the majority of children today are functioning with optimal detoxification systems.

In *Nontoxic, Natural, and Earthwise*, Debra Dadd indicates the extent to which chemicals have permeated our bodies and our lives. She cites a study done by the EPA in which 100 percent of the people tested had styrene, xylene, 1-4-dichlorobenzene, ethylphenol, and dioxin in their adipose (fat) tissue. Additionally, 96 percent had benzene, 91 percent had toluene, 83 percent had PCBs, and 55 percent had DDT. These toxic chemicals only represent a fraction of chemicals found stored in these individuals.

I think these statistics are even more important when we evaluate whether or not our children's detox systems are functioning optimally. I have yet to find a study that proves that children do not have these kinds of chemicals stored in their bodies to the same extent that adults do. In contrast, I have read many studies which prove that children are actually *more* likely to have toxic chemicals in them. These studies show that children are more at risk to suffer adverse effects from chemical exposures because 1) the amount of toxins they inhale from the air or ingest per pound of body weight is greater than adults, 2) their cells divide more rapidly, 3) they have some immature organs that absorb toxic chemicals more readily, and 4) they have lower levels of the enzymes required for detoxing.

Unfortunately, I believe that many children are already showing the symptoms of a dysfunctional detox system, but because most people do not understand the detox system, their symptoms are either being treated with medications (which might only further damage the system) or are being passed off as the behaviors of a "naughty" child. While I realize that it is no one's intent to purposely harm these children, in a sense, it almost seems like a form of child abuse to continue to medicate or punish children who really just need to have their dysfunctional detoxification systems properly treated.

Opposition

Hopefully, this book has helped convince you that the chemicals in our lives *do* impact our health. But be prepared to encounter a whole slew of people who will disagree with you.

Unfortunately, even family members of individuals who have impaired detox systems may dismiss the whole affair as nonsense. At the detox clinic, it was not uncommon to hear of spouses or parents who did not believe their husbands, wives or children were really sick. In some ways, this is not surprising. These family members may have never heard of environmental illness before ("she's reacting to the carpet—WHAT???"). They might have believed environmental illness really existed if their own trusted doctor had made this diagnosis. But, instead, many of their family doctors told them that "there is no such thing" as environmental illness.

In such cases, I think it is imperative that people first understand that the educational training of most doctors does not include any information about environmental illness or about the body's detoxification system. Furthermore, most doctors are not trained to recognize the symptoms of an impaired detox system. If an illness does not match up with symptoms listed in traditional medical textbooks, many doctors conclude that the illness must have an emotional or mental basis. This is the way they have been taught to think. Consequently, it is not surprising that many of the leading doctors in environmental medicine are those who became environmentally ill themselves (or had a family member who did) before they changed their medical practice. Many of these doctors on the front line of environmental medicine are labeled "quacks" by their colleagues (which is not unusual when a doctor deviates from the norm).

At one point during my illness, I had to confront the traditional medical community when the state required that I see one of its own physicians if I wanted to continue receiving my disability checks. I certainly was not very thrilled about this since I figured that the chance of the state physician having any understanding of environmental illness was almost nil.

But since the requirement came after I had been to the detox clinic, I at least knew what was wrong with me, and I had copies of the blood tests that indicated my chemical toxicity. However, as I waited for the state's doctor to enter the examining room, I feared that my badly needed checks were on shaky ground. Moreover, I was certainly not relieved when, referring to the possibility that daily chemicals can cause illness, the first words out of this doctor's mouth were, "You know all of this is very controversial."

I agreed with her, but then I looked her straight in the face and said, "But, unfortunately, it is no longer controversial to *me*." I then asked her how she as a doctor dealt with medical controversy. My question made her acknowledge the possible scenarios which might occur if certain controversial ideas discarded by a doctor are proven correct in the future.

Just when I thought she was coming around, she looked at the copies of the blood tests I had brought and actually said, "These don't mean shit."

When I asked her to explain, she agreed that the tests did show that there were elevated levels of toxic chemicals in my bloodstream. But she did not agree that the tests *proved* that the chemicals were making me sick (though her conclusion is obviously not shared by all doctors). When I asked what sort of proof she would need, she sort of stumbled and didn't really answer. I then asked her if she thought a sickness only occurred after the testing for it had become perfected. In other words, was she implying, for example, that no one had had cancer until the biopsy was perfected?

Her facial expression conveyed that she thought these were valid questions. After a somewhat long discussion, I am happy to report that the doctor recommended that the state continue my disability checks.

However, I realize that this small victory will probably still not prompt other doctors, major manufactures, pest control companies, or even government agencies to change their emphatic claim that the chemicals in our lives are not harming us. Occasionally, someone will tell me that his or her doctor has told them that patients who claim to have a long list of unrelated symptoms resulting from chemicals are, in truth, hypochondriacs. Sometimes I think people tell me this just to see my reaction. But, I usually just laugh and shake my head. After all, I'm sure there were many people in Columbus's day who still claimed the world was flat even after he returned from his voyage—especially if their livelihood depended on making maps of flat worlds.

CEREBRAL ALLERGIC REACTIONS (TOXIC BRAIN SYNDROME)

Chemicals can affect any part of the body, including the brain. Whereas a reaction in the lungs might trigger asthma, a reaction occurring in the central nervous system might trigger changes in a person's thought, perception, motor control, and behavior.

My first experience with a cerebral allergic reaction (or toxic brain syndrome) made my daughter's stuffed purple pony legendary in my family. However, before I tell this story, I want to first point out some characteristics of my behavior prior to my becoming chemically sensitive so you can see how the chemicals dramatically changed my behavior.

Before I became ill, it would certainly be fair to say that I had become angry on occasion. However, I was never known to slam a door, hurl an object, or resort to tantrums to express my anger. Instead, I was the type who would articulate my perspective, point by point, and then follow the targeted person around (just ask my husband) until he or she finally acknowledged my viewpoint. However, when I had cerebral reactions, my behavior completely changed.

At the time of the purple pony incident, I had not yet learned about chemical sensitivities, let alone cerebral reactions. I only knew that the major sinus surgery, which four doctors had told me would help me breathe better, had actually left me worse off than before. Looking back, I now know that the physical stress from the surgery, the general anesthesia (which produced a horrendous forty-eight hour adverse reaction in me) and the intravenous, round-the-clock antibiotics I was taking had all combined to sink me deeper and deeper into chemical overload and ill-health. But at the time, all I knew was that I was still sick. Enter the infamous purple pony.

Still very weakened from surgery and my "mysterious" illness, I was lying on the couch one evening when I asked my husband to make a phone call for me. He responded that he would. But as I waited, I saw him doing other things. When I asked again, he said he would do it later.

LATER!!! An incredible, illogical surge of anger overcame me. When I once again asked him to make the call right then, he again responded that he would do it later.

I cannot even begin to explain the anger I was feeling. I had never experienced anything like it before. I felt like he had betrayed me in the worst possible way. So, when I spotted my daughter's purple stuffed pony at my side, I quickly grabbed it and threw my hand back in position to throw—and maim.

My husband looked at me, unconcerned. Nothing in his fifteen years of knowing me prepared him for the purple pony smacking him in the face moments later! In addition to never thinking that I would throw the pony, he never imagined that in my weakened condition I would be able to hit a bull's-eye!

Since that episode, I have unfortunately had other cerebral reactions (my husband has since learned to duck when he recognizes what is happening). Of all my diverse symptoms from allergic reactions—dizziness, swelling of the throat, shortness of breath, and so on—these cerebral reactions remain the most devastating to me. While I am not in physical pain during a cerebral reaction, the mental anguish of being so out of control is more horrendous to me than any physical symptom.

My friends, who have never witnessed one of my cerebral reactions, tell me that they cannot imagine me screaming, pulling my hair, or sobbing hysterically (some of my behaviors during the worst reactions). In fact, after the reaction has subsided, even *I* cannot believe my behavior. But, there is nothing I can do to prevent the illogical anger or the incredible depression that overcome me during a cerebral reaction any more than I can loosen my throat when it has swelled or walk straight when I am dizzy. These behaviors are all allergic reactions to something, and the brain is not excluded from being a sensitive organ.

Not surprisingly, as I continue to get better, these cerebral reactions occur less frequently since I now avoid chemicals that I know trigger reactions in me, and I am repairing my detoxification system. In fact, at the moment, I cannot recall when I last experienced a major cerebral reaction. Now I usually have comparatively minor episodes in which either my motor control is affected (whereby I either keep dropping things or can't even read my own handwriting), or I experience a mild mood swing.

You might be wondering how I and other people who have suffered from toxic brain syndrome differentiate between true anger or depression and the anger or depression resulting from a cerebral reaction. Or you may think that *everyone* has days when they drop things or write sloppily.

However, remember that the brain is a primary target of toxins. Through my own experiences and those I know who also suffer from cerebral reactions, I can share some of the common factors that indicate a cerebral reaction is the cause of the behavior change.

First, with cerebral reactions, there appears to be *no logic* to the person's behavior change. For example, I would never cry or get hysterical when my throat swelled, my chest burned, or my stomach became nauseous. However, as soon as the major physical symptoms subsided, I would sometimes become illogically depressed or angry. In fact, I can remember a time when I was having such a severe breathing attack that I wasn't sure I was going to make it. But as I lay on the bed, I was motivated to "hang on" because I was determined to stay alive for my girls. But as soon as the breathing attack subsided, I remember suddenly feeling depressed, hopeless, and worthless and thinking that my girls would be better off without me. I even told my husband that it would be better if I just died. After all, the girls were young, he was smart and attractive, and they would all just be better off without me. These wild mood swings made no sense to me until I finally understood toxic brain syndrome.

Furthermore, a cerebral reaction causes you to blow things out of proportion. For example, my husband might toss his jacket on the couch and leave it there. The next morning, if I am not having a cerebral reaction, the jacket's presence on the couch might still bother me a little. I might shake my head or sigh out loud. However, if I am having a cerebral reaction, you would think that he had dumped the entire contents of his closet on the couch by the way I reacted. During a cerebral reaction, his jacket becomes THE ENEMY. My rage is so out of proportion that it is almost unbelievable. What is worse is that I am aware of what I am saying (or, more accurately, yelling), but I JUST DON'T CARE. During a cerebral reaction of this kind, it is as if my voice has become disconnected from my heart or soul—or even worse. It is like demons have temporarily entered my body, turning me into someone entirely different. As soon as the reaction passes, I am mortified by the scene I have created (especially when I think about the trivial cause that prompted such behavior).

I know that it is also very difficult to be around a person who is having a cerebral reaction, especially since there is really nothing you can say or do to alleviate the horrible mental anguish the chemically sensitive person is experiencing. (My husband once made the unfortunate error of making me even angrier by saying, "Oh, you're just having a cerebral reaction.") It is also difficult because neither family members nor the chemically sensitive person ever knows when or what kind of cerebral reaction is coming.

At the detox clinic, I had the opportunity to watch other people have cerebral reactions. It was common for patients to have them as they were detoxing the numerous chemicals stored in their bodies. I especially remember when this one man, who was the nicest, funniest, and most well-liked person at the clinic, had a cerebral reaction. I could hardly believe what I witnessed. All the nurse did was ask him how long he had been out of the sauna. This was something she asked the patients all the time since it was part of her job to make sure that, generally, people did not take longer than ten minute breaks.

In the past, he would just joke with her when she asked this. However, on this particular occasion, he became LIVID. He started to verbally attack her. Not only was he yelling loudly, but he was using locker room language (every other word) to make sure that she understood that HE would decide when HE was ready to get back in the sauna.

Becoming aware that cerebral allergic reactions exist can change a person's life. One woman at the detox clinic had always thought she had severe emotional problems because she experienced panic attacks whenever she was in a crowd of people. But after making the cerebral connection, she realized that she was not afraid of people; rather, she reacted to their clothing, perfume, and shampoos.

I have a friend whose sister became intrigued by a Phil Donahue show about cerebral reactions in children. Prior to watching this show, the mother had become convinced that her adopted daughter's extreme, negative behaviors (tantrums, violent hitting, throwing, biting, etc.) and emotional problems were the result of her unfortunate past and her being adopted as an older child. The mother had arranged counseling for her daughter, but, thus far, the sessions had not brought about any improvement.

But after watching the Donahue show, the mother began to consider whether or not cerebral allergies might be affecting her daughter. She located a physician trained in this area and made an appointment.

Allergy testing proved that certain foods—not her past—were actually responsible for this little girl's extreme behaviors. When the offending foods were eliminated from her diet, it was as if a complete personality change overcame the child. As long as she avoided the foods she did not experience cerebral reactions. At the next family reunion, my friend noted that it did not even seem to bother the six-year-old that she had to eat differently. Despite the fact that she was only six, she completely understood the negative effect certain foods had on her and had absolutely no desire to eat them.

In contrast to all the other children who may unknowingly suffer from cerebral reactions, I believe that this little girl is one of the lucky ones. She now knows that she is not a naughty, horrible, mean little girl. Instead, she realizes that she is merely a girl who experiences cerebral reactions when she eats certain foods.

Cerebral Reactions at School

I often find myself thinking about all those children whose negative behavior might unbeknownst to them be triggered by adverse reactions to chemicals. Likewise, what about all those compassionate teachers and parents who, despite patience and discipline, cannot help a child who is unmotivated or who just goes berserk at times? At least I had thirty-four years of "normal" behavior against which I could compare my cerebral reactions; thirty-four years worth of normal behavior showed that the irrational behaviors I exhibited during cerebral reactions were not "me." In fact, because my cerebral reactions were so out-of-character, they prompted us to search for some physical, medical explanation for them. But what about those children who may not have the same baseline for comparison that I did—those children who have been reacting to environmental triggers since birth or early childhood?

Since I used to be a teacher, I started wondering specifically how cerebral reactions might be affecting student behavior and academic performance at school. As I started learning about toxic brain syndrome, I began to think about past students of mine. Almost immediately, a student named Laura came to mind.

Laura was the one student I had who I could never seem to get motivated. While she never demonstrated negative behaviors, she frustrated me because she would just sit all of the time as if in a daze. (When she did move, it was at the pace of a turtle.) She expressed interest in getting her work done, but she never did. Even though I had no knowledge at that time of toxic brain syndrome, I had wondered if drugs were somehow responsible for her behavior. (She was only ten and I found no evidence to confirm drug use.) Laura remained a mystery to me.

Given what I know now, I'll bet anything that Laura was experiencing cerebral reactions. She had all the physical characteristics of an allergic child (to be discussed shortly). In fact, I met a patient at the detox clinic whose behaviors reminded me EXACTLY of Laura. It took hours for this patient to finish a sentence, and she seemed to be in a fog all of the time. I was never sure how she even found her way from the dressing room to the saunas.

But after just three weeks at the detox clinic the change in this patient was incredible. It was no longer torture to have a conversation with her. In fact, the more she detoxed, it became evident that she was actually a very bright and witty woman. I found myself wishing even more that I had known about cerebral reactions when Laura was in my class.

After watching my own improvement and learning about environmental triggers, my sister, who is a fifth grade teacher, could not help but apply some of this new information to the students in her class. For example, she had one student who had been pegged as having a "behavior" problem. A thick file documenting occurrences during his previous five years of schooling verified this label.

But as my sister became more familiar with some of the signs of chemical reactions, she noted that this student had several of them. She began to suspect the possibility of a chemical problem even more when she observed an undeniable change in this student's behavior after the class had worked on an art project using bleach. This prompted her to tell him about some of my experiences with chemical reactions.

I later went to her classroom for a visit. At lunch time, rather than playing with his friends, the boy chose to stay in and talk to me about chemical reactions. He asked me countless questions about how chemicals could suddenly change someone's behavior. When I told him there was a book by a pediatrician who worked daily with children with cerebral reactions, he quickly ran to his desk for a pencil and paper and asked me to write down the name of the book.

Throughout our entire conversation, I felt saddened as I watched this ten-year-old become elated over the possibility that there might actually be a reason for his extreme behaviors. It was as if a tremendous burden was being lifted from his shoulders to know that the negative, disliked side of his personality might not really be his fault.

I do not know what eventually happened to that student. The next school year he transferred to another school. I would love to say that the child ran home and told his parents about our conversation, and they immediately began to search for a doctor trained in environmental medicine to either rule out or confirm the role of chemicals in their son's behavior.

But, unfortunately, that is probably not what happened. I know of other parents of "problem children" who have been given this same information but who chose to do nothing to help their children. I can only conclude that these parents must so strongly accept the myth (perpetuated by many doctors, commercial enterprises, and the government) that the chemicals in our lives are harmless, that they find it easier to accept having a problem child than having a child who is sensitive to chemicals and/or food.

Certainly, not all negative behaviors are prompted by chemical reactions. Children do throw temper tantrums because they are angry. Children do become cranky because they are tired. But some children do exhibit extreme behaviors because they are having adverse reactions to environmental triggers. It is a fact.

Documented studies show a direct correlation between allergic reactions and both hyperactivity and learning difficulties in children. I think the connection between allergic reactions and hyperactivity is very significant considering that 75 percent of prisoners in jail today were hyperactive children.

Dr. Crook, a leading pediatrician who focuses on environmental medicine, conducted a study on forty-five children who suffered from either hyperactivity or learning difficulties. The results of his study are remarkable. Food allergies were the cause of symptoms in *forty-one* of the forty-five children. The symptoms were either partially or totally relieved when the offending food(s) were no longer eaten. (For those children whose symptoms were only partially relieved, other chemical testing may be warranted.) The children were generally allergic to three foods. Twenty-eight of the forty-five were sensitive to milk. Other common offenders were sugar, eggs, wheat, and corn.[7]

Dr. Rapp, another well-known pediatrician specializing in environmental medicine, has occasionally found that IQ test scores may improve after proper allergy treatment. After just six months of allergy treatment focusing on diet and environmental changes and allergy extract therapy, a four-year-old patient of Dr. Rapp no longer spat, bit, hit, or wildly threw his toys. But even more amazing was the improvement in this boy's score on the Wechleser Preschool and Primary Scale of Intelligence (WPPSI). Prior to beginning allergy treatment, the boy scored 81 on the Verbal IQ (low average), 99 on the Performance IQ (average), and 88 on the Full Scale IQ (low average). After six months of allergy treatment, he scored 109 on the Verbal IQ (average-above average), 110 on the Performance IQ (average-above average), and 110 on the Full Scale IQ (average-above average).[8]

Allergies have also been linked to autism, mental illness, and juvenile delinquency. In many cases, appropriate allergy care has greatly reduced some or all of these negative behaviors. The implications of this, not just for children but for society as a whole, are staggering.

Doctors practicing environmental medicine do not believe that *every* physical symptom or negative behavior is the result of an allergic reaction to something in the environment. But they do consider the possibility that environmental triggers can cause symptoms and affect behavior. If it weren't for these doctors, many children might end up with labels such as juvenile delinquent, slow learner, inattentive, or aggressive or continue to have chronic health problems through adulthood while never making the cerebral reaction/dysfunctional detoxification system connection.

EAR INFECTIONS

At any given time, it seemed that more than half of the children in my daughter's play group were on antibiotics for another ear infection. The moms would comment that we never recalled having so many ear infections when we were young. But we never pursued the question of why so many young children today seem to have recurring ear problems.

I now know that there are four major causes of fluid build-up in the ear—allergy, infection, mechanical obstruction, and nutrient deficiency. Regardless of the different causes for this fluid, the term "ear infection" is generally used by both doctors and parents. However, to always call fluid build-up in the ear an ear *infection* may be incorrect. The medical term for this condition, otitis media, means ear *inflammation*—not infection. This difference may be very important when considering that most ear infections are treated with antibiotics even though antibiotics will not reduce inflammation. In fact, in approximately 30 to 50 percent of cases of otitis media, the children *do not* have harmful bacteria in the middle ear. This may explain why many children's ear problems do not respond to antibiotics.

Moreover, repeated use of antibiotics may actually contribute to recurring ear problems. Antibiotics can weaken a child's overall health condition by eliminating "good" intestinal flora. This, in turn, can cause intestinal yeast (Candida) to multiply, resulting in a chronic health condition. While most traditional doctors recognize Candida as a local infection (e.g., oral thrush and vaginal yeast infections), other doctors acknowledge that Candida, as a chronic health problem, can cause multiple symptoms, including allergies. (Recall that allergies are one of the causes of otitis media.) Giving a child repeated rounds of antibiotics may further burden the child's detoxification system—especially if his or her detox system is already impaired.

Considering that before antibiotics were introduced, approximately 80 percent of all ear problems were spontaneously cured, parents may begin to question whether or not every ear infection needs to be treated with antibiotics. Furthermore, parents should consider the possibility that allergies, mechanical obstruction, or nutrient deficiency might be the cause of their child's ear "infection."

FOOD SENSITIVITIES

Traditional allergists insist that food allergies only occur in those persons who have *fixed* reactions. A fixed reaction is when a person will always have a reaction if he or she eats a certain food—even if he or she has not eaten the food for years. It is estimated that only a few people out of every thousand actually have fixed food allergies.

In contrast, it is estimated that 60 percent of the population has some kind of food *sensitivity*.[9] Food sensitivities, which may develop over time, are adverse reactions to a food or a drink. Many traditional allergy doctors do not believe that food sensitivities exist because the skin testing they rely on to prove a food allergy may or may not prove a food sensitivity.

However, doctors specializing in environmental medicine, as well as other doctors, recognize that people can become sensitized to food. There are three types of reactions caused by food sensitivities: cumulative reactions (which occur only after eating a certain amount of the food or after eating the same food several times in a short period of time), variable reactions (which occur without any logical pattern), or addictive reactions (which occur if a person does not eat a food he or she craves).

One way a person can become sensitive to a food is by eating the same food every day. Another way is by having Candida overgrowth in the intestines. When a Candida overgrowth occurs, thereby creating a condition in which there are more bad bugs in the intestines than good, digestion and absorption of nutrients becomes poor, and the gut wall of the intestines becomes irritated and inflamed. As a result of this irritation and inflammation, large molecules of food are able to cross the intestinal border and enter the bloodstream. When this happens, the body then begins to make antibodies against the molecule resulting in symptoms such as abdominal pain, distended abdomen, gas, coughing, chest pain, asthma, swollen throat or tongue, fatigue, diarrhea, mood swings, heart palpitations, and bed-wetting.

Common foods that children can be sensitive to include: wheat, dairy products, citrus fruits, corn, and sugar. In one study of 1,000 patients, milk, chocolate, cola, corn, citrus fruits, and eggs were found to be the most common offenders. In this study, milk was the number one offender for children under the age of two. In addition to these foods, food coloring and additives have also proven to cause a variety of symptoms.

Most people have probably never considered that bed-wetting might be an allergic reaction. Bed-wetting usually causes much embarrassment for a child, especially an older child, and a bed-wetting child may eventually need counseling. Yet, interestingly, food sensitivities to milk, fruit juices or fruit (especially raisins), or other foods can trigger bed-wetting. In one case study, a child who had been wetting his bed for nearly *six* years stopped after oranges were removed from his diet.

There is an explanation for how bed-wetting is affected by allergies. When a person eats a food to which he or she is sensitive, the muscular coating around the bladder contracts. This makes the bladder smaller and keeps it from holding normal amounts of urine. The result can be more urination during the day and bed-wetting at night. Additionally, a drug-like sleep sometimes follows the ingestion of a problem food, which then results in a child simply not waking up when the bladder signals that it is full.

Each person's response to a food sensitivity is going to be different since each person's biochemistry is different. The type of reaction a person experiences will also depend on how well that person's detoxification system is working at the time. That is why no one can say that a particular food (or chemical) will cause the same symptom for everyone or will cause the same symptom in a person every time.

Food allergies (versus chemical allergies) can be suspected when symptoms and behaviors do not seem to follow any pattern. For example, a parent might note that there is no change in symptoms and/or behavior if the child is indoors, outdoors, at home, or at school. Even if food is suspected, it may be difficult to determine which food is causing the problem because processed foods often contain *many* ingredients. Additionally, even when a food has been identified as causing problems for an individual, it may still be difficult to eliminate that food. Parents must remember to carefully scrutinize the ingredients of processed foods.

For example, let's imagine that an infant is sensitive to corn. The mother avoids giving her child corn, but she does not notice that the formula she gives her baby contains corn syrup. (Corn syrup is a very common ingredient in many products.) The baby may have reactions to the corn syrup, act fussy, for example, without the mother ever making the connection. She may even change formulas. But she will probably just buy another one with corn syrup since she has overlooked this ingredient before. Breast-fed babies may also demonstrate symptoms of food sensitivities if their mother's milk contains traces of a food that the baby is sensitive to.

In addition, people may be sensitive to *several* foods. Relief from symptoms may not occur until all foods that cause problems for an individual have been identified and eliminated.

It is also important to keep in mind that symptoms from food sensitivities do not necessarily occur right after the food is eaten. This makes it difficult for many to accept that a food is causing the symptoms. Such was the case with a friend of mine whose son complained of recurring stomach cramps and burning. When I mentioned the possibility of exploring food sensitivities, the idea was dismissed since my friend saw no obvious connection between her son's stomach problems and his eating habits.

Instead, the three-year-old child underwent extensive blood testing and an upper GI to determine if the child had an ulcer or any other major stomach problems. The tests did not reveal anything. The doctor told her that everything was fine, but her son still had the pains.

The doctor now had two choices. Fortunately for my friend and her son, instead of recommending that the boy undergo counseling, the doctor decided to look at the foods the boy ate. It turned out that apple juice (which the boy drank daily) was causing his stomach pains. When apple juice was removed from his diet the stomach pains stopped. When the apple juice was re-introduced, the symptoms returned.

I am not suggesting that there is never a reason to do extensive blood work or upper GIs. But when one considers both the mental and physical stress of these tests (not to mention the cost), they might not be the most appropriate first step for diagnosing stomach pains. If elimination diets or provocation-neutralization allergy testing (to be discussed shortly) show nothing, then sophisticated tests for an ulcer (which is quite rare in a three-year-old) or other stomach conditions is, of course, warranted. But not the other way around.

SOLUTIONS AND ALTERNATIVES

Hopefully knowing how to identify and repair a dysfunctional detox system will make the information presented in the problem section of this chapter seem not quite as overwhelming.

SIGNS AND SYMPTOMS OF AN ALLERGIC CHILD

I used to say that I never had an allergy problem until my downfall with pesticides and chemicals. However, in researching for this book and in the process of learning more about allergies, I have come to the conclusion that I did, indeed, demonstrate signs of mild allergies since childhood. As a child, I had numerous nose bleeds for no apparent reason and infrequent episodes of shortness of breath. In my later years, it seemed that every time I returned to my parents' home for a visit, I caught the flu or a cold. Back then, my family used to joke that I just waited to get sick at home so that Mom could take care of me.

However, I now know that my parents' house contains a tremendous amount of mold, to which I am extremely sensitive. Mold can be found in many unsuspecting places. It can grow in carpets, duct work, worn clothing, air conditioners, books, plants, pets, litter boxes, and some other unlikely places. In addition, mold spores in the air that we cannot see can easily be inhaled.

While hives and sneezing may be obvious signs of allergies, there are also many less-known signs of an allergic child. These symptoms might also signal a dysfunctional detoxification system. The common physical signs include glassy, glazed eyes; red ear lobes; dark blue, black, or red circles under the eyes; red, rouge-like cheeks; wrinkles below the eyes; nose wrinkle (from rubbing the nose upwards); and unexplained facial pallor.[10] It should be noted that not all of these symptoms may be present or need to be to confirm an allergy. Many of these symptoms will also appear and then disappear.

Some common behavior signs of an allergic child include sleepiness, spaciness, fidgetiness, lapses in concentration, inattentiveness, hyperactivity, depression, fatigue, loudness, silliness, and illogical anger.[11] Rapid speech, stuttering, and imitating animal sounds have also all been associated with allergies.

Unfortunately, I have experienced most of these symptoms at one time or another. To help you understand how these symptoms can affect a chemically sensitive person's life on a daily basis, I will share some of my own experiences. However, keep in mind that another person with a different biochemistry and different detoxification system might respond differently.

SLEEPINESS It is almost guaranteed that I will begin to feel drowsy if I am caught in a traffic jam. Hydrocarbons cause me to appear as if I have been sedated with sleeping pills. Fortunately, the few times that this has happened, I was not driving. (I am happy to say that since I purchased a car air filter, I no longer have this problem.)

INATTENTIVENESS I can recall times when no matter how much I would try to follow a conversation, I just could not comprehend what the other person was saying. I would watch the person's lips move and hear the voice, but for the life of me, I could not tell you what she was talking about.

DEPRESSION I can remember a time when I thought of taking a kitchen knife and cutting my hand because I thought the physical pain from the cut would have to supersede the indescribable mental anguish I was experiencing. Fortunately, I have always maintained a thread of sanity during my cerebral reactions which has prevented me from doing anything self-destructive. However, I recently read of a chemically sensitive person committing suicide.

MOTOR CONTROL There are times when it seems as if I drop or knock over everything in sight. Sometimes this is my only sign that I am having a cerebral reaction to something.

INTOLERANCE TO SUNLIGHT Prior to becoming sick, I was in the sun as often as it shone. Now, it is impossible for me to be outside for even a few minutes without my large, white visor (which has since earned me the nickname the "Flying Nun.")

INTOLERANCE TO NOISE During my days of intense detoxing at the clinic, I was so sensitive to noise and sounds, that I could not be in a room with more than a few people at a time. Even now when I am having a reaction, noise seems to quadruple in volume.

INTOLERANCE TO ODORS AND AN ACUTE SENSE OF SMELL I used to swear that I could smell pesticides residues from our pest control sprayings days after everyone else claimed the air had "cleared." I could also tell you when someone was lighting a barbecue down the street. I almost could tell you your toast was burning before it had even turned black.

Many substances in the home may cause these and other symptoms: aerosols, ammonia, bleaches, carpet glues, dust mites, feathers, floor cleaners and waxes, formaldehyde (which is in such things as adhesives, concrete, fabric, mouthwashes, nail polish, furniture, and paper products), fungicide-treated wallpaper, gas stoves and appliances, hair sprays, insecticides, molds, newspaper print, oven cleaners, paint fumes, pesticides, pets, pine-scented cleaners, plastics, room deodorizers, scented soaps, shampoos, and synthetic clothing.

Outside the home, the following have been known to trigger allergic reactions: grass, weeds, pollens, wet leaves, insecticides, aerial chemical sprays, fresh asphalt, and factory pollution.

In the schools, the troublemakers include: art supplies (paint, marking pens, glues), chalk, perfume scents of the teacher, mimeograph or chemically-treated paper, fluorescent lamps, and portable classrooms (which typically contain formaldehyde, glues and other toxic materials). In addition, the exhaust fumes from the school bus may trigger a reaction in a child before he or she even gets to school.

New Allergies

It is important to remember that since the body has the ability to adapt to the stresses placed on it, symptoms from an allergy may not actually appear for some time. Some parents may rule out the possibility that their child has allergies simply because their child has never previously shown allergic symptoms. I would like to stress that until I became sick two years ago, I had not exhibited any of the bizarre physical or behavior symptoms I describe. But almost overnight I became a person with countless allergies. (Of course, now I realize that this occurred when I had reached the threshold point and my detox system began its downward spiral.)

If your doctor does not understand an impaired detoxification system, he or she may not be willing to accept the notion that your child suddenly has developed allergies—especially if the symptoms are not the ones generally associated with allergies.

For example, at the onset of my illness, I went to the emergency room because I was experiencing great difficulty in breathing. Additionally, my left eyelid was swollen, I was weak, and I was urinating excessively despite the fact that I had not been drinking fluids. When the ER doctor asked me what was wrong, I blurted out (in between gasps for air) that I thought I was having an allergic reaction to something. Even though I knew of no allergies at that time, it just intuitively seemed that I was having an allergic reaction.

But when the ER doctor then asked me if I had any known allergies or asthma, I, of course, responded no. Well, that was that. With the look that I was going to become accustomed to over the next six months, he then wanted to know why I "thought" I could not breathe. And since a chest x-ray showed nothing (as may be the case in an allergic reaction), I was sent home again to the house that had just been oversprayed with pesticides.

Testing For an Impaired Detox System

There are blood tests that can help determine the condition of someone's detoxification system. Different blood panels test for decreased levels of glutathione peroxidase, elevated levels of lipid peroxides, depressed levels of sugar oxide dimsultase, increased mercapturic acid and/or D-glucaric acid, and an elevated level of formic acid. Each of these tests relates to a specific function of the detox system. The results of these tests are considered indicators of a problem, rather than absolute proof of an impaired detox system.

Not all labs perform these tests. However, your physician can send your blood to Monroe Labs in Southfields, New York; Doctor's Date in Chicago; or National Medical Services in Willow Grove, Pennsylvania, to have these tests done.

According to Dr. Rogers, the formic acid test can be done in any doctor's office. This test determines how well your body is handling aldehydes (but reveals nothing about other detox pathways). If the level of formic acid in your blood is too high, Dr. Rogers says "you're like an accident waiting to happen."

A high level of formic acid (which is a metabolite of formaldehyde) in the blood signifies a backlog of formaldehyde in the detox pathways. This indicates that your detox system is not successfully getting rid of it fast enough. This backlog of formaldehyde places an additional burden on the entire detox system. Therefore, any additional exposures to chemicals, such as from a new carpet, will likely trigger a multitude of adverse reactions.

Provocation-Neutralization Testing

Provocation-neutralization testing is when a patient is given a small diluted extract of a food, chemical, mold, or fungi. The extract is either injected in the arm or placed on the tongue. After the dose has been given, any reactions to the substance (physical or behavioral) are monitored. This testing is used to identify which environmental triggers are causing problems and what antigen can be administered to cancel the symptoms.

Many traditional allergists do not believe in this type of testing. However, these doctors cannot explain how a tiny drop of allergy extract can cause a variety of symptoms in a patient, including changes in the person's handwriting. Doctors who use provocation-neutralization testing can also show how allergy extracts can cause dramatic mood swings. Doctors have numerous examples of nice, friendly pictures drawn by young children prior to their being given an extract to which they are allergic, as well as examples of violent, angry pictures drawn by the children after they were given the extract.

In addition to my own experience, I have seen fascinating video tapes of children undergoing provocation-neutralization testing. One tape showed a two-year-old, who was completely calm before he was injected with an allergy extract, throw a temper tantrum moments after he was injected. Critics who claim the child started screaming because of the prick of the needle cannot explain why the child suddenly calmed down when he was injected with the neutralizing antigen.

I have also seen examples of incredible changes in handwriting as a result of someone having an adverse reaction to a substance. At the detox clinic, the patients daily recorded their symptoms on charts. If you reviewed the charts, you would notice dramatic changes in the patient's handwriting on those days of intense detoxing.

While provocation-neutralization testing can be used to determine which substances cause adverse reactions in an individual, people can also be administered routine shots (or drops) of neutralizing antigens as part of an allergy treatment program. Many allergy sufferers have noted significant improvement with this approach.

DETECTING FOOD AND CHEMICAL SENSITIVITIES

According to Dr. Doris Rapp, one simple way of determining if sugar, food coloring, or additives are causing reactions in your child is to throw a party for your child and his or her friends. When the young guests first arrive, ask them to write their name or draw a picture.

Forty-five minutes after you serve the party food (cookies, cake, ice cream, punch) again ask them to write their name or draw a picture. If you notice any changes in the writing/drawing, or if you notice any changes in behavior (e.g. aggressiveness, silliness, withdrawal), then the children may be reacting to the sugar they just consumed. Also observe if the children have bright red earlobes, glassy eyes, or dark circles under their eyes, as these are also symptoms of a food sensitivity.

Skeptics might say that the changes in the children's behavior were due to the mere excitement of the party. To disprove this, invite the same children to a party at which you only serve vegetables. If the children do not exhibit the same changes in behavior, you can be even more assured that the sugary, artificially colored and flavored foods prompted the behavior changes at the first party.

Without really intending to implement this type of test, I had the opportunity to see the results with the children in my girls' play group when the group had its annual Christmas party. The food at the party consisted of traditional, sugar-laden Christmas goodies.

About midway through the party, I noticed that all of the children, except my own, were either running, screaming, fighting or crying. I am not implying that my children never run, scream, fight, or cry. But, unlike the rest of their friends, they were doing none of these things at the party. Additionally, the other children in the playgroup did not normally act this way either.

There was only one difference between my girls and the rest of the children at the party. My girls had not eaten any of the party treats. I concluded that it was not the excitement of Santa's arrival and the festivities that had prompted the behavioral changes in the other children. Rather, it appeared to me that the combination of the sugar, food coloring, and additives in the party food *and* the holiday merriment had been too much stimuli for most of the children.

Different diets can be effective in determining if your child suffers from food sensitivities. These include the Single Food Diet, the Multiple Food Diet, and the Rotary Diet (which is both diagnostic and therapeutic). All of these diets can be followed at home. Both Dr. Crook's book *Tracking Down Hidden Food Allergies* and Dr. Rapp's book *The Impossible Child* provide detailed explanations of the diets and outline how to implement them.

The Parent Detective

Parents may have to become detectives in order to determine what environmental triggers may be causing problems for their child. Parents can first try to determine if a pattern exists to their child's reactions and exposures to specific substances. However, this is not always that easy.

First of all, reactions do not always occur immediately after an exposure—they can sometimes occur as long as twenty-four hours later. Therefore, it may be difficult to identify if the reaction was triggered by something the child was exposed to at school or at home. It may even be something the child was exposed to yesterday. Additionally, the child may not react identically to the same incitant all of the time. (Remember, how a body reacts to a substance will depend on what pathways are open in the detox system.)

Another crucial concept parents must understand when playing detective is that of "total overload." For example, it may be that your child has a slight sensitivity to milk and is also allergic to ragweed. Until ragweed season, your child might be able to drink milk without experiencing any reactions. But as ragweed season approaches, the *combination* of these two factors might cause him or her to have symptoms. Additionally, many food-sensitive people have noted that they can eat certain foods in the summer, but not in the winter. Some of these same people complain of having a "cold" all winter long.

In such a situation, one might suspect the home furnace. Furnaces create more air turbulence, stirring up more dust and mold spores, which are both very common allergic incitants.

If your home has a gas furnace, then it may be the gas itself that is the problem. For the longest time, we could not figure out why my symptoms always seemed to get worse at night. It seemed like as soon as the sun went down, so did I.

However, during one unusual week in February when it was so warm we did not need to turn the furnace on at night, I felt significantly better. After a few nights of consistently feeling better, we began to suspect the furnace. On the first night we turned the heat on again, I expected that my symptoms would once again intensify. However, this did not happen. (This is why detective work can be very frustrating, especially if one does not understand the total overload theory.) But shortly thereafter, the old pattern returned, and I once again felt worse at night. A visit to my parent's home a few weeks later confirmed that I have adverse reactions to gas.

In contrast to my mostly-electric home (the exception being the heating system), my parents' home is all gas. On this particular visit one cold, rainy morning, my mother simultaneously had on her gas dryer, gas washer, gas oven, and gas furnace. Needless to say, I was practically comatose. When we figured out what was happening (it always seems so obvious after the fact), I chose to sit out in the freezing rain until the house could be aired out.

Here are some specific steps that parents can take to help figure out what might be stressing their children's detox systems:

1) Find out what times of the year that tree, grass, or weed pollens are most evident in the local area. Note if there is any pattern between symptoms and times of the year.

2) If a child mentions or complains about smelling odors, try to identify where the smell is coming from (however, the odor may be very faint or not even be noticeable to a person who is not chemically sensitive). Try to determine if there is any relationship between this source and the child's physical symptoms and/or negative behavior.

3) For suspected sources of allergic reactions, put the item (e.g., cleaning fluid, polyester fabric, moldy fruit) inside a glass jar. Tighten the cap and leave it on for at least thirty-six hours. (For fabrics, some physicians recommend placing the jar in a warm area.) Then, open the jar and have the child sniff the contents. Some individuals have an immediate reaction (e.g., a

headache, nausea, nasal congestion) while others (delayed reactors) may not show symptoms until later. (For these individuals, the sniff test will have to be repeated in order to determine whether or not the tested item was the indeed the trigger.) If no symptoms occur, then the child is probably not allergic to the item.

4) Keep a record of what a child eats and note if any foods seem to trigger symptoms.

Without question, the body is a complicated machine. Parents are most successful in determining food and chemical sensitivities if they are working in conjunction with a medical doctor trained in environmental medicine. This partnership works best because parents are in the position to observe daily occurrences, while the doctor is in the position to provide guidance and testing to confirm or rule out suspected offenders.

Allergies and School

One of the guidelines for recommending that a student undergo special education testing is teacher observation of specific discrepancies in the child's academic performance. For example, if a student is an outstanding reader, but cannot seem to add even the simplest computation, a teacher might suggest the child be tested. But what if, for example, the child is unknowingly sensitive to milk and he drinks milk every day at lunch? And what if math is only taught AFTER LUNCH? It might be that the student has trouble with math because every afternoon he suffers an adverse reaction to the milk he had for lunch, not because he has a learning disability.

Also, consider what might happen if a child is tested for a learning disability right after he or she has eaten a food or been exposed to a substance to which he or she is sensitive. Certainly, the person administering the tests may indeed see abnormalities. But do the test results show that the child has a learning disability or that the child may be having an allergic reaction to a food or a chemical? I know that I would hate to be tested for anything when I am having a reaction.

With all the cost, extensive testing, and documentation required to place a child in special education classes, it seems that ruling out environmental factors should be a mandatory part of the evaluation process. Likewise, with all the time and energy devoted to students who have behavioral problems, it also seems logical to test whether or not environmental factors are the cause of their problems as well.

A special group of parents and teachers can be formed to help others become aware of the possible link between chemical exposures and learning and/or behavior problems in students. The group can encourage the school or district to purchase video tapes which are available through the Practical Allergy Research Foundation (see Appendix 2). These tapes clearly demonstrate the impact chemicals commonly found in schools can have on sensitive children. Even if your own child does not appear to have symptoms, identifying the problem of another child in the classroom can actually help your own child. When a teacher has to spend extra energy on the "problem" child in the classroom, all students inevitably suffer.

NATURAL APPROACHES FOR TREATING EAR INFECTIONS

Both of my girls got their first ear infections when they were approximately three months old. Thereafter, they continued to have recurring ear infections, all of which were treated with numerous rounds of antibiotics. The doctor even discussed surgically placing tubes in the ear of my youngest to drain fluid. However, by the time the tubes were recommended, I had already become skeptical of traditional medicine's enthusiasm for "fixing" a symptom without first identifying the *source* of those symptoms.

At that time, I had not yet learned about chemical and food sensitivities, but I had read two books, written by medical doctors, about Candida as a chronic health condition. In addition I had read numerous testimonies from pediatricians, including Dr. George Shambaugh, the former president of the American Academy of Otolaryngology, about how children who had suffered from repeated ear infections experienced positive results after being treated for Candida. Then I learned that milk products are the main food allergy associated with ear infections. I found myself thinking about all of the dairy products my daughter's consumed, including three glasses of milk a day (as prescribed by their pediatrician) as well as all the antibiotics they had taken.

Therefore, when the pediatrician said that our daughter had yet *another* ear infection, we decided to forgo the traditional antibiotics. Instead, we were determined to try some alternative approaches. As recommended by my acupuncturist, we gave our daughter some homeopathic ear drops (containing mullein and garlic oil) and a homeopathic remedy (chamomilla). We also immediately eliminated from her diet fruit, dairy products, and all food containing yeast or sugar. We were willing to wait at least twenty-four hours to see if these alternative treatments were working. After all, we could still fill the prescription if she seemed worse.

When the pediatrician phoned the next day to see how my daughter was doing, and I casually mentioned that we were considering not filling the prescription for antibiotics, I received a long speech about how not treating ear infections with antibiotics could be life-threatening. Even my own parents looked at us doubtfully as my little girl's fever climbed to almost 104 degrees.

But twenty-four hours later, she was undeniably improving. The next day she was even better, and on the third day she was fine. Ten days later, we returned to the doctor's office to verify that the ear infection had indeed cleared. In the past, this was when the doctor usually told us that the ear was "still a little infected" and then gave us a prescription for more antibiotics. But this time—for the first time—after examining our daughter the doctor said, "Beautiful! Clean as a whistle!"

Based on this success, we decided to eliminate all dairy products and refined sugar from our children's diet and limit the amount of fruit and yeast products they consumed. We had become convinced that allergies were playing a significant role in our daughters' ear infections.

Our intuition appears to have been correct. During the past two years, my eldest daughter has had no ear infections, and my youngest has had just one. In the past, they usually had between five and eight ear infections each year. While we believe that dairy products and sugar were the primary causes of our daughters' ear problems, some other common foods that have been linked to recurring ear problems include eggs, soy, shellfish, wheat, chocolate, and corn. Common airborne offenders are cigarette smoke, formaldehyde, pollen, carbon monoxide, mold, and household dust. To learn more about the causes of recurring ear problems and alternative treatments, read *Childhood Ear Infections*, by Michael A. Schmidt. It is an excellent, informative resource.

REPAIRING YOUR CHILD'S DETOX SYSTEM

If chemical exposures can stress a child's detox system, it follows that reducing chemical exposures will help repair the stressed system. Therefore, to ensure that your child has a functional detoxification system, I highly recommend that furniture, building materials, personal care items, toys, art supplies, baby products, and any other products that have been made out of toxic chemicals, as well as pesticides, herbicides, and fungicides, be eliminated as much as possible from your child's life. I also highly recommend including organic produce, legumes, and whole grains in your child's diet since the nutrients found in these foods are key to the detoxification process.

I realize that we cannot control everything that our children will be exposed to. But I also know that if we reduce their toxic exposures by creating a nontoxic home and by providing them with a diet based on organic whole foods, there is a much better chance that their detox systems will be able to handle the toxins that they encounter when they venture out into the world.

Teaching Your Child

Over the course of our family's lifestyle changes, my girls have occasionally been referred to as junior Ralph Naders. Some people are amused that such young children have an awareness of toxins and chemicals; however, others have made the comment a bit disparagingly. It's nothing personal, Ralph. I understand the tongue-in-cheek tone used by my friends and acquaintances since it was not that long ago that environmental and consumer issues were not top priority in my life either.

Ralph Nader presents a paradox to many people. On the one hand, these people are certainly thankful that there is someone "watching out for us." But on the other hand, there is a subconscious fear that Ralph (or others) may uncover something that would mandate changes in their present lifestyles. Change seems to frighten most people.

Additionally, some people have implied that we have been teaching our children to live in fear. This criticism was also made against parents who boycotted apples during the Alar scare of 1989. According to the critics, parents were causing psychological damage by making their children afraid to eat apples.

However, this same criticism is not hurled at parents when they teach their child how to cross a street safely (e.g., cross at corners, look both ways, wait for a green light). To emphasize the importance of being cautious when crossing a street, parents usually explain what can happen if the child is not cautious. However, nobody says the parent is instilling in the child an unreasonable fear of streets. Teaching children about the dangers of toxins in the world is no different from teaching them about the dangers of not being cautious when they cross a street.

A Lesson

It was important to me that my children understood that it was *multiple* chemical exposures combined with a certain lifestyle that had damaged my dysfunctional detox system and triggered my illness. To illustrate this point, I presented a simple demonstration using a piece of typing paper.

I held up the paper and began naming all the toxic things that I had consumed or been exposed to in the past—refined sugar, processed food, sprayed produce, pesticides, cleaning chemicals, new carpets, and so on.

As I named each exposure, I made a small rip in the paper to represent the impact that it had had on my body. As I tore the paper more and more, my girls could not help but notice that it no longer looked like the same white sheet of paper.

After numerous tears, we then tried to predict when the paper would fall apart. But we did not have a sure method for determining this. So I continued naming toxins and ripping the paper until, finally, the paper was no longer one, complete sheet.

As my girls watched the first torn piece fall to the ground, I explained that the human body was not much different. It certainly was strong enough to take a rip here and there, but it was very difficult to predict how many rips a body could endure before it would "fall apart."

But I also wanted my girls to recognize the incredible healing powers of the human body. So I proceeded to show how we could try to piece the paper back together again. Using scotch tape, we slowly started taping each piece of paper. The task took us quite a long time. Once we finished, while we concluded that the taped paper was now "functional," we unanimously agreed that it was still not the same nor as strong as it had once been.

This exercise helped illustrate how long it takes to heal a dysfunctional detoxification system and the possibility that the body may never be as strong as it had once been. It also refuted the sometimes cocky (perhaps subconscious) attitude of those who believe that whatever may go wrong with the human body can be fixed by a doctor or a drug. (I cannot tell you how many people have asked me, "Isn't there something you can just take?")

In conclusion, I asked my girls if we had been given any prior warning that the paper was going to fall apart. After thinking about it, my girls agreed that if we had stopped ripping about midway, the paper probably would have never become completely torn. They also concluded that had we started piecing the paper back together much earlier, then it would have been a lot easier to restore.

I explained to them that the body, too, gives us warnings and signs. One of my first complaints to my doctor (several months prior to my becoming seriously ill) was excessive perspiration. I was perspiring for no apparent reason—even in cold weather. Of course, I now know that my poor body was making one last ditch effort to rid itself of the toxins I kept exposing it to. But back then I just was told to buy a stronger (chemical) deodorant.

From a Child's Perspective

As a result of our family's experience with natural healing, our two preschool children have become very intuitive about their own bodies. In fact, they have actually come to believe that their bodies "talk" to them. As my oldest clarifies, "Of course, my body doesn't know words, but it still can tell me things."

For example, now if she eats too much fruit and her face breaks out in a rash, she concludes that her body is telling her "enough." When she is tired and cranky, instead of fighting going to bed, she now understands that her body is just telling her that it needs sleep.

She has even extended this new awareness to health conditions among her friends. One day she surprised me by casually commenting, "You know, Mom, Amy's body has been talking to her, too."

Amy was her friend who every winter caught a lingering cold. Recently, I had concluded that poor diet and/or other environmental factors might be the cause of this little girl's ill health, but I had never told my daughter this. So, when my daughter stated that "Amy's body was talking to her," I was very intrigued.

"How do you know that?" I asked.

"Well," my daughter replied, "you know all those colds and runny noses she always has." And then, in a very resigned voice, she sighed, "But I can't tell her. She'll just have to find out for herself."

One day my daughter amazed me even more with her insight. Throughout all our conversations about health and bodies and changes, I was never quite sure how much of it my children internalized. However, on this particular day, my daughter showed me that she did understand what we had been teaching her by using a word that had never come up in any of our conversations about the human body.

She turned to me with a sparkle in her eye and said, "Mommy, my body is magical."

I was astonished. No, I was flabbergasted. In one short sentence, she expressed what I had been trying to teach her over several months.

Yes, she saw that the body was not invincible; I was proof of that. But given a chance to function as intended—without being constantly bombarded with countless daily chemicals and toxins—she also recognized the body's magical power to heal itself. I was proof of that, too. But more importantly, she had internalized this at the mere age of three.

Without question, our new lifestyle is not the norm. However, now upon hearing a tongue-in-cheek Ralph Nader reference or some other comment alluding to the fact that we may be psychologically damaging our children by making them so "different," we usually just smile.

We smile because we are not concerned about what these critics say. We know that our children's primary lesson has not really even been about chemicals or a new diet. Instead, what they have truly come to understand is the concept of cause and effect. And what they have begun to appreciate is that there is freedom in this country for individuals to acquire knowledge and to live accordingly.

My daughters do not think this makes them different; they believe it makes them special.

IN THE FUTURE

Sometimes, it may seem that my discussion of chemicals is exaggerated. But it bears repeating that your children and mine are not living in the same world we grew up in. Perhaps if toxins had been gradually introduced into our lives then the human body might have had a chance to gradually adjust to them. But they were not.

Just think about what the average child is exposed to today. One cannot even begin to count the chemical and artificial substances that invade our daily lives. Additionally, our children were exposed to chemicals the minute they were born; they were never given the chance to grow up in a clean, healthy environment. When looking at the situation from this perspective, it does not seem preposterous to conclude that chemicals may greatly impact the health of our children. In fact, it seems preposterous to insist that they do not.

I am aware that upon finishing this book you may feel somewhat overwhelmed. Without question, I have presented a lot of information. And, if you are anything like I was just two years ago, the information is both new and mind-boggling.

But I want to take this last opportunity to reassure you. Even though I do hope that individuals will be motivated to make some changes in their lives, I will not be disappointed or discouraged if some people don't make any changes right away. I feel this way because I think that just reading the information presented in this book changes people.

You will be different after reading this book because you will know about the chemicals in our lives. What you ultimately decide to do with this knowledge—either now or in the future—is your personal choice. And that choice is to be respected—as long as it does not directly infringe upon the health of others.

I also know that different individuals need different time periods to absorb and then apply new information. For example, I have two friends with children who have now been identified as having adverse reactions to chemicals and/or food. Both friends knew the information in this book for almost a year before they finally decided to act upon it. But, while it may have taken them a year to implement the necessary changes, the beginning of their change occurred when they first were exposed to this information.

Individuals (like myself) with chemical sensitivities have had to make dramatic, immediate changes in their lifestyles simply because they suddenly found themselves unable to remain healthy in a chemical world. While some may still not find our situation applicable to themselves, others have likened us to canaries in a coal mine. (This refers to when miners took canaries down into the coal mines with them to warn them when the air became too bad—the miners got out when the canaries died.) Some believe that persons with multiple chemical sensitivities today are like society's canaries, warning those yet to be affected.

Obviously, it is my most sincere hope that all parents will begin to acknowledge the undeniable relationship between chemicals and health. Unquestionably, it is a sad song that some of us "canaries" are singing today, but it will become an even sadder song if no one listens.

But I refuse to conclude this book on a note of pessimism. This book is not about doom. When I look back at all I have experienced in the past two years, this book is a celebration to me. It is a celebration of how knowledge can be so powerful that it can enable individuals, like myself, to become well again. This book is a celebration of families and friends, proving the incredible positive impact that love and support can have. It is a celebration of personal freedom, showing that individuals do have the right to choose what they put inside their bodies and surround themselves with. It is a celebration of social commitment since many individuals, publishers, businesses, organizations, and doctors, are already dedicated to educating and helping others acquire this important knowledge and make the necessary changes. Last of all, this book is really a celebration of life itself, complete with its surprising turns and challenges—all of which I am very grateful to still be experiencing.

CHECKLIST FOR SUGGESTED CHANGES
AND COMMITMENTS

☐ Ensure that your child's detoxification system is working optimally by reducing his or her exposures to chemicals (see chapters 2, 3, and 5) and by providing meals of organic whole grains, legumes, and vegetables (see chapter 4).

☐ If warranted, find a clinical ecologist in your area who can assist you in identifying what possible substances may be affecting your child.

☐ Purchase an audio cassette about environmental illness that tells you how to conduct various allergy diets and how to make your home more allergy- and chemical-free. (Tapes are available from the Practical Allergy Research Foundation, P.O. Box 60, Buffalo, NY 14223-0060.)

☐ To determine whether or not your child may have sensitivities to certain substances or foods, observe any relationships between exposures and symptoms, place your child on an elimination diet (consult *Tracking Down Hidden Food Allergies* by Dr. William Crook), or have provocation-neutralization testing done on your child.

☐ Form a group of parents and educators to increase awareness of the impact that chemical exposures can have on behavior, learning, and overall academic performance.

☐ Teach your children about the impact of toxic chemicals as you use nontoxic alternatives.

APPENDIX 1

Recommended Further Reading

HOME

Dadd, Debra. *Non-toxic, Natural and Earthwise.* Los Angeles: Jeremy P. Tarcher, Inc., 1990.

Bond, Anne Berthold. *Clean and Green: The Complete Guide to Nontoxic and Environmentally Safe Housekeeping.* Woodstock, NY: Ceres Publishing, 1990.

Graff, Debra. *Pest Control You Can Live With.* Steerling, VA: Earth Stewardship Press, 1990.

Roussea, David. *Your Home, Your Health, and Well-Being.* Berkley, CA: Ten Speed Press, 1988.

ENVIRONMENTAL MEDICINE/ALLERGIES

Crook, William, M.D. *Tracking Down Hidden Food Allergies.* Jackson, TN: Professional Books, 1978.

Crook, William, M.D. *The Yeast Connection.* New York: Random House, 1986.

Golos, Natalie and Frances Golbitz. *Coping With Your Allergies.* New York: Simon and Shuster, Inc., 1979.

Rapp, Doris, M.D., and Dorothy Bamberg, *The Impossible Child.* Buffalo, NY: Practical Allergy Research Foundation, 1986.

Rogers, Sherry A., M.D. *Tired or Toxic?* Syracuse: Prestige Publishing, 1990.

Schmidt, Michael A. *Childhood Ear Infections: What Every Parent and Physician Should Know about Prevention, Home Care, & Alternatives.* Berkeley: North Atlantic, 1990.

FOOD

Duffy, William. *Sugar Blues.* New York: Warner Books, 1976.

Garland, Anne Witt. *For Our Kids' Sake.* New York: National Resources Defense Council, 1989.

McEntire, Patricia. *Mommy-I'm Hungry.* Sacramento, CA: Couger Books, 1985

Oski, Frank, M.D. *Don't Drink Your Milk.* Syracuse, NY: Mollica Press, 1983.

Turner, Kristina. *The Self-Healing Cookbook.* Grass Valley, CA: Earthtone Press, 1987

APPENDIX 2

Resources

Note: The resources are listed by general categories. A listing in this appendix does not constitute an endorsement of the product, company, organization, or person. Rather, this information has been included to show you the many resources available for nontoxic living. Since many of these companies offer multiple items, the same company may be listed more than once, and I have not listed every item that a company sells. Most of the companies offer free catalogs. I encourage you to order the catalogs to learn more about the companies and *all* of their products.

SPECIFICALLY FOR CHILDREN

After the Stork
1501 12th Street NW
Albuquerque, NM 87104
(800) 333-5437
Offers a wide variety of children's clothing made from natural fibers.

Autumn Harp
28 Rockydale Road
Bristol, VT 05443
(802) 453-4807
Offers talc-free baby powder, petroleum-free jelly, petroleum-free baby oil, and baby shampoo made from plant oils and herbs.

Baby Bunz and Company
P.O. Box 1717
Sebastopol, CA 95473
(707) 829-5347
Offers a wide range of natural diapering products, including Nikkys and Dovetails; 100 percent cotton clothing

for infants; wooden baby rattles and dolls made from all-natural materials; lambskin booties; lambskin blanket.

Biobottoms
Box 6009
3820 Bodega Avenue
Petaluma, CA 94953
(707) 778-7945
Offers diapers, diaper covers, diaper duck for soiled diapers, an "It's easy to diaper with cloth" starter kit, 100 percent cotton clothing and shoes.

Cot'nKidz
P.O. Box 62000159
Newton, MA 02162
(617) 964-2686
Offers natural fiber clothing with standardized sizing and accessories for infants to ten years.

Country Comfort
28537 Nuevo Valley Drive
P.O. Box 3
Nuevo, CA 92367
(800) 462-6617
Offers natural baby powder, oil, and cream.

Earth's Best Baby Food
P.O. Box 887
Middlebury, VT 05753
(800) 442-4221
Offers a selection of organic baby foods and cereals.

Family Clubhouse
6 Chiles Avenue
Asheville, NC 28803
Offers a complete diapering system, which includes the Dovetail for those times when a disposable is necessary.

J.R. Liggett, Ltd.
Route 12-A
RR2 Box 911
Cornish, NH 03745
(603) 675-2055
Offers J.R. Liggett's Old Fashioned Bar Shampoo (which contains natural ingredients to help eliminate head lice).

Motherwear
P.O. Box 114
Northampton, MA 01061
(413) 586-3488
Offers 100 percent cotton clothing for infants and toddlers; wool blankets and changing pads; handcrafted toys, 100 percent cotton bouncer seat; 100 percent cotton baby carriers; natural diapering products, including Bumpkins all-in-one diapers; baby care products made from natural ingredients; and a nontoxic insect repellent for children.

National Association of Diaper Services
2017 Walnut Street
Philadelphia, PA 19103
(800) 462-6237
Can assist you in finding a diaper service in you area.

Natural Baby Company
RDI, Box 160
Titusville, NJ 08560
(800) 388-BABY
Offers diapers, including Nikkys; diaper covers; baby care products; disposable diapers that have no dioxin, plastic or chemicals; lambskin rugs; wool blankets; hardwood rattles; a line of wooden toys, soft dolls, and wooden furniture that "can be handed down to your grandchildren."

Natural Lifestyle Supplies
16 Lookout Drive
Asheville, NC 28804
(800) 752-2775
Offers natural diapering products; toys made from natural materials and non-toxic paint; and a baby gift set which includes a wooden shaker rattle, Weleda baby care, travel size baby soap and cream, Earth Child baby powder, one dozen cloth diapers and two decorative Nikky diaper covers.

Papa Don's Toys
Walker Creek Road
Walton, OR 97490
(503) 935-7604
Offers toys made from natural materials.

Perlinger Naturals
238 Petaluma Avenue
Sebastopol, CA 95472
(707) 829-8363
Offers a selection of baby foods which come from biodynamic farms (Biodynamic farming is called the "cream of organic farming" since the guidelines for it are the strictest in the world.)
These baby foods contain no sugar, salt, fillers, binders, modified starches, or preservatives.

Seventh Generation
49 Hercules Drive
Colchester, VT 05446
(800) 456-1177
Offers talc-free baby powder, baby
soaps, comforters and crib sheets made
from dioxin-free 100 percent cotton
fiber without dyes or formaldehyde,
dioxin-free baby wipes made with
lanolin and no alcohol or artificial scent,
and petroleum-free jelly.

Simply Pure Food
RFD #3, Box 99
Bangor, ME 04401
(800) 426-7873
Offers organic strained and diced baby
foods as well as organic baby cereals.

WeCare
77-725 Enfield Lane, Suite 120
Palm Desert, CA 92260
Offers watercolors made from plant
concentrates, colored pencils free of
heavy metals and wrapped in untreated
cedar, and crayons made from natural
waxes and earth pigments.

NONTOXIC PEST CONTROL

Brody Enterprises
9 Arlington Place
Fair Lawn, NJ 07410
(800) 458-8727
A family owned and operated pest control firm for over fifty years. Claims to
have the largest catalog of poison-free
pest control products. Offers traps,
repellents, and more.

EcoSafe Products, Inc.
P.O. Box 1177
St. Augustine, FL 32085
(800) 274-7387
Offers natural flea control products,
natural diatomaceous earth, and an insect repellent made of herbs in a natural
base that works against mosquitos,
fleas, and flies.

Flea Busters/Rx for Fleas
Flea Busters are located in Alabama,
California, Connecticut, Delaware, Flor-
ida, Georgia, Hawaii, Louisiana,
Maryland, New Jersey, North Carolina,
Ohio, Oregon, South Carolina, Texas,
Virginia, Washington D.C., and Wash-
ington state. Call (800) 666-3532 for the
name of a Flea Buster distributor in your
area.

A Flea Buster service person will come to
your home and apply a completely nontoxic, odorless, fine white powder
(which is primarily a mineral salt compound) to your carpet. The active ingredients is sodium polyborate which,
according to the company, "is no more
harmful than table salt." The Flea Buster
powder is effective against fleas because
it makes the carpet an environment less
conducive to fleas. A one-year guarantee
is offered; the product is EPA registered.

Nontoxic Termite and Ant Control
(800) 543-5651
Will refer you to a local pest control
company that uses the electrogun
method (instead of pesticides) to
eliminate termites. The electrogun is also
effective against powderpost beetles and
carpenter ants.

Perma Proof
1929 W. Howard Street
Chicago, IL 60626
(312) 764-5559
Offers natural pest products and management services in Chicago and surrounding suburbs. Additionally, the
company sells an odorless product to kill
roaches, ants, silverfish, and waterbugs.
All services and products are backed by
a written guarantee.

Safer, Inc.
189 Wells Avenue
Newton, MA 02159
Offers a wide variety of products for
controlling specific pests. Also found in
most health food stores and garden
shops.

Whole Earth Access Company
2990 7th Street
Berkeley, CA 94710
(800) 845-2000
Offers natural pet products.

PESTICIDE-FREE WOOD

Floyd Shelton Superior Floors
500 3rd Street, Suite 326
Wausau, WI 54401
(800) 247-4705
Offers oak floor planks that have never
been treated with any pesticides.

GENERAL MULTIPURPOSE NONTOXIC COMPANIES (Paint, Sealants, Finishes, Adhesives, Polishes, Cleaning Products, Cosmetics, Personal Care Products, Household Items, Test Kits, etc.)

AFM Enterprises
1440 Stacy Court
Riverside, CA 92507
Offers nontoxic paints, sealants, carpet
guards, waxes, adhesives, shoe polishes,
tile grout, and spackling compound.

Baubiologie Hardware
The "Healthful" Hardware Store
200 Palo Colorado Canyon Road
Carmel, CA 93923
(800) 441-8971
(408) 625-4007
Offers products for a healthier, safer
home free of hazardous toxic chemicals.
Has materials such as natural linoleum,
nontoxic adhesives, nontoxic paints,
ozone machine, air filters, and electromagnetic shields and aprons. Also of-

fers formaldehyde, water and air test
kits.

The Living Source
3500 MacArthur
Waco, TX 76708
(817) 756-6341
Distributor of a wide variety of nontoxic
products such as personal care products,
cosmetics, air filters, household items,
fabrics, cleaning products, Odor-Fresh
(zeolite), and building materials.

Livos Plantchemistry
1365 Rutina Circle
Santa Fe, NM 87501
(505) 438-3448
Manufactures products such as paints,
plant-based cleaners, stains, varnishes,
adhesives, floor wax, liquid furniture
wax, soap made with natural ingredients
as well as low-toxic building supplies.

N.E.E.D.S.
120 Julian Place
Syracuse, NY 13210
Offers a wide variety of items for a nontoxic lifestyle such as books, air and
water filters, cleaning products, cosmetics, and full spectrum lights.

Nigra Enterprises
5699 Kanan Road
Agoura, CA 91301
(818) 889-6877
Distributor of nontoxic products such as
air purification systems, water purification systems including shower attach-
ments, room heaters, vacuums, interior
and exterior paints, upholstery sealants,
wood stains, tile grout, caulk, waxes,
cleaners, and mold retardants.

Pace Chem Industries, Inc.
779 S. LaGrange Avenue
Newbury Park, CA 91320
(805) 499-2911
Offers products which contain no
petrochemicals or toxic ingredients.
Pace's Crystal Aire protects and en-

hances all woods (cabinets, furniture, paneling, etc.), plasterboard, colorfast wallpaper, vinyl and clay tile, paint and other finishes. As a sealant, Crystal Aire blocks out formaldehyde and other toxic fumes. Pace's Crystal Shield is a durable nontoxic hardwood floor finish which dries in just two hours. It also blocks out formaldehyde and other toxic fumes.

Sinan Company
P.O. Box 857
Davis, CA 95617
(916) 753-3104
Offers natural building materials which contain no petroleum base, crude oil, or plastic ingredients. Offers varnishes, lacquers, wall paints, adhesives, and art supplies. In the company's free catalog, each product has a comprehensive listing explaining how the natural product works and application recommendations.

Seventh Generation
(See address under "Specifically for Children")
Offers nontoxic household cleaners, dishwashing liquids, polishes, unbleached (dioxin-free) paper, animal repellent, shower filters, personal care products, 100 percent cotton towels and bedding that are unbleached and undyed.

Sunrise Lane
780 Greenwich Street
New York, NY 10014
(212) 242-7014
Offers nontoxic body lotions, skin care products, conditioners, shampoos, hair coloring, household cleaners, make-up, nail care products, soaps, suntan lotions, toothpaste, and perfumes made from pure plant extracts in alcohol-free and grain alcohol base.
Lifetree, a product line of Sunrise Lane, offers a dishliquid, an all-purpose household cleaner, a premium laundry liquid, an automatic dishwashing detergent, and a home soap.

VAPOR BARRIER

E.L. Foust Co., Inc.
Box 105
Elmhurst, IL 60126
(800) 226-9549
Offers Dennyfoil Vapor Barrier which meets FHA requirements for vapor protection on floors, sidewalls, and ceilings. It is also effective against mildew and dampness. No petroleum products, fire retardants, mold retardants, pesticides, or formaldehyde are added to Dennyfoil during the production process.

NATURAL FIBERS (Cotton and Silk)

The Cotton Place
P.O. Box 59721
Dallas, TX 75229
Offers 100 percent cotton bedding, batting, clothing, needlework supplies, and fabrics.

The Janice Corporation
198 Rt. 46
Budd Lake, NJ
Offers 100 percent cotton bedding, towels, clothing, shower curtains, and throw rugs.

Motherwear
(See address under "Specifically for Children")
Offers 100 percent cotton flannel nursing pajamas, night gowns and night shirts, and fashion wear designed for the nursing mother.

Winter Silks
2700 Laura Lane
P.O. Box 130
Middleton, WI 53562
(800) 648-7455
Offers silk sweaters, long johns, sleepwear, and fashions.

AIR AND WATER PURIFICATION

E.L. Foust Co., Inc.
(See address under "Vapor Barrier")
Offers air and water filters.

Environmental Purification Systems
P.O. Box 191
Concord, CA 94522
(800) 829-2129
Created by a person with chemical sensitivities. Offers products designed for those with environmental illness as well as those who have become aware of the daily health hazards associated with air and water contaminants. Products include a shower filter, a whole house air filter, room air filters, and whole house water filters.

G & W Supply
1441 W. 46th Avenue #31
Denver, CO 80211
(800) 738-6343
Offers Odor-Fresh, the trade name for zeolite, the natural mineral that absorbs smoke, bacteria, and some indoor air chemical contaminants.

Memphremagog Heat Exchangers
P.O. Box 456
Newport, VT 05855
(802) 334-5412
Offers a heat recovery ventilation unit.

Mia Rose
1374 Logan, Unit C
Costa Mesa, CA 92626
(714) 662-5465
Offers a natural, non-aerosol spray to freshen rooms and reduce airborne viruses, bacteria, and smoke. It is also an effective pest repellent.

Riehs & Riehs
501 George Street
New Barn, NC 28560
(919) 636-1615
Offers a heat recovery ventilation unit.

LIGHTING

Baubiologie Hardware
(See address under "General Purpose Nontoxic Companies")
Offers a radiation-free fluorescent bulb. This bulb eliminates virtually all flicker associated with other kinds of fluorescent lamps.

Nuclear Free America
325 East 25th Street
Baltimore, MD
(301) 235-3575
Manufactures bulbs which contain no radioactive material and no mercury. Ecoworks bulbs use 10 percent less energy than standard incandescent bulbs and last three times as long.

MATTRESSES AND BEDDING MADE OUT OF ORGANIC COTTON OR UNTREATED WOOL

Bright Future Futon
3120 Central Avenue SE
Albuquerque, NM 87106
(505) 268-9738
Offers organic cotton futons in all sizes as well as yoga exercise mats, traditional Zen meditation pillows, and other pillows.

Dona Designs
825 Northlake Drive
Richardson, TX 75080
(214) 235-0485
Offers futons (including crib size), innerspring mattresses, mattress pads, pillows, and comforters made form organic cotton and covered with unbleached cotton.

Pure Podunk, Inc.
Podunk Ridge Farm
RRI Box 69
Thetford Center, VT 05075
(802) 333-4256
(800) 776-3865
Offers 100 percent untreated wool mat-

tresses, futons (including crib size), comforters, mattress pads, pillows, and handspun yarns made of wool from sheep raised on a small New England farm. Covers are made with untreated cotton and sewn with linen thread. For information on how to apply for financial aid for Pure Podunk products, write the company.

NONTOXIC CLEANERS AND DETERGENTS

Bon Ami Company
Faultless Starch/Bon Ami Co.
1025 West 8th Street
Kansas City, MO 64101
Manufactures a scouring powder that does not contain chlorine.

Ecover (Mercantile Food Co.)
4 Old Mill Road
P.O. Box 1140
Georgetown, CT 06829-1140
Offers products which do not contain phosphates, bleaches, enzymes, petroleum detergents, NTA or EDTA (which have both been identified as being carcinogenic) or synthetic dyes or coloring. Ecover offers laundry powder, wool wash liquid, floor soap, and non-chlorine bleach, toilet cleaner, liquid laundry soap, and dishwasher powder.

Granny's Old-Fashioned Products
P.O. Box 256
Arcadia, CA 91006
(818) 577-1825
Offers products which are EDTA and petroleum free including an all-purpose liquid soap, a laundry detergent, and a carpet shampoo. Soaps are made with coconut oil surfactants.

NONTOXIC COSMETICS AND PERSONAL HYGIENE PRODUCTS

Aubrey Organics
4419 N. Manhattan Avenue
Tampa, FL 33614
(813) 876-4879
($3.00 for catalog, but most products can be found in health food stores.) Offers soap, shampoos, cosmetics which are made from vegetable sources. Products contain no perfumes, artificial colors, or preservatives.

Country Comfort
(See address under "Specifically for Children")
Offers pure herbal salves and natural lip cream sticks.

Desert Essence
P.O. Box 588
Topanga, CA 90290
(213) 455-1046
Offers natural products using pure Australian Tea Tree Oil such as toothpaste and mouthwash.

Dr. Bronner's
All-One-God-Faith, Inc.
Escondido, CA 92015
Offers natural soaps and pure castile liquid soap.

Ecco Bella
125 Pompton Plains Crossroads
Wayne, NJ 07470
(800) 888-5320
Offers cosmetics, moisturizing creams, and lotions.

Paul Penders
1340 Commerce Street
Petaluma, CA 94954
Offers natural hair care, skin care and make-up products.

Tom's of Maine
Railroad Avenue
Kennebunk, ME 04042
Manufactures shampoos, including coconut-based shampoos that contain no preservatives, artificial dyes, or animal ingredients; 100 percent aluminum -free deodorant; and a shaving cream made of olive oil and other natural ingredients.

Real Purity Cosmetics
The Living Source
(See address under "General Multipurpose Nontoxic Companies")
Offers cream foundation, lipstick, blush, mascara, eye shadow, and sunscreen made from natural ingredients.

DIOXIN-FREE PRODUCTS

C.A.R.E. (Consumer Action to Restore the Environment) Products
(Ashdun Industries, Inc.)
1605 John Street
Fort Lee, NJ 07024
(201) 944-2650
All products are made from a chlorine-free bleaching process and are made entirely from recycled fibers. Products include paper towels, toilet paper, facial tissue, napkins, coffee filters, cotton swabs, and cotton balls.

✓ **Earth Care Paper Company**
100 S. Baldwin
Madison, WI 53703
(608) 256-5522
Offers unbleached writing paper of every kind, holiday cards, wrapping paper, and envelopes.

✓ MAIL ORDER ORGANIC FOOD

Note: Many of the companies listed below ship their perishables in a styro-lined box with ice packs for proper insulation. Both the boxes and the ice packs are recycled by issuing a call-tag

with UPS which has UPS automatically return to the home within a day or two to pick up the box at no extra cost to the customer.

Brandon Sea Pack
P.O. Box 5488
Charleston, OR 97420
(800) 255-4370
Offers glass packed salmon and tuna with no additives, except sea salt if requested.

French Meadow Bakery
2610 Lyndale Avenue
Minneapolis, MN 55408
(612) 870-4740
Makes breads from organic grains without dairy products or yeast.

✓ **Gold Mine Natural Food Co.**
1947 39th Street
San Diego, CA 92102
(619) 234-9711
(800) 475-3663
Offers organic grains, beans, nuts, pastas, sweeteners, as well as traditional macrobiotic foods. Also publishes the *Gold Mine Gazette* which contains articles and a listing of products.

Green Earth Natural Foods
2545 Prairie Avenue
Evanston, IL 60201
(800) 322-3662
Sells organically grown produce; organic meat and poultry (meaning that in addition to no growth hormones or antibiotics being given to the animal, the animal was fed organic feed); organic cheeses; soy cheeses; organic breads (including bagels); organic juices; organic teas; organic grains; organic oils; soy milk; coffee substitutes; non-dairy yogurt; and biodynamic eggs.

Mountain Ark Trading Company
120 S. East Avenue
Fayette, AR 72701
(800) 643-8909
Offers organic products that include
produce, grains, legumes, cereals, grain-
sweetened candy, oils, condiments,
pastas, teas, beverages, sea vegetables,
and other macrobiotic foods.

**Natural Beef Farms Food Distribution
Co.**
4399-A Henninger Ct.
Chantilly, VA 22021
(703) 631-0881
Offers organic beef, chicken, pork,
lamb, veal, lunch meats and cheese and
yogurt made from organic milk. Also
sells fresh produce, frozen produce,
entrees, side dishes, breads, grains,
cereals, chips, snacks, spreads, syrups,
soups, spices, beans, pasta, pickles, coffee, and juices, all of which are organic.

Natural Lifestyle Supplies
(See address under "Specifically for
Children")
Offers organic and macrobiotic specialty
foods. Also offers natural grain-
sweetened candy with no artificial coloring or flavorings.

Organic Foods Express
11003 Emack Road
Beltsville, MD 20705
(301) 937-8608
Offers fruits, vegetables, flours, grains,
nuts, and beans.

Walnut Acres
Penns Creek, PA 17862
(717) 837-0601
Offers cereals, flours, grains, baked
goods, soups, oils, peanut butter, canned
and dried vegetables.

MILK SUBSTITUTES

Mountain Ark Trading Company
(See Address under "Mail Order Organic Food")
Offers a variety of flavors of soy milk.
Also sells Rice Dream, a delicious non-
dairy beverage made from organic
brown rice. Rice Dream can be served
hot or cold and comes in vanilla and
chocolate flavors.

SWEETENER SUBSTITUTES

Gold Mine Natural Food Co.
(See address under "Mail Order Organic
Food")
Offers amaske, barley malt, and rice
syrup.

Lundburg Family Farms
P.O. Box 369
Richvale, CA 95974
(916) 882-4551
Offers barley malt and rice syrup along
with other organic foods.

Wax Orchards
22744 Wax Orchard Road SW
Vashon, WA 98070
(800) 634-6132
Offers products made from a blend of
natural concentrated natural fruit juices
for baking or cooking. Products also
come with recipes.

SOME HEALTH FOOD COM-
PANIES FOUND IN HEALTH
FOOD STORES

Arrowhead Mills	Erewhon
Bronner	Health Valley
Chico-San	Lima Oshawa
De Sousa	Nature's Path
Desert Gold	Shiloh Farms
Eden	Westbrae

ORGANIZATIONS

American Academy of Environmental Medicine
P.O. Box 16106
Denver, CO 80216
Offers a listing of medical doctors throughout the country trained in environmental medicine. Send $3.00 and a self-addressed, stamped envelope for a listing for your area.

Americans For Safe Food
1501 16th Street, NW
Washington, DC 20036
(202) 332-9110
A large coalition of groups promoting contaminant-free food. Publishes a comprehensive list of mail order organic food companies.

Bio-Integral Resource Center (B.I.R.C.)
P.O. Box 7414
Berkeley, CA 94707
A non-profit organization which provides information on least-toxic pest control management. Publishes an annual directory of safe pest control products and services.

Center for Safety in the Arts
5 Beekman Street
New York, NY 10038
(212) 227-6220
Distributes books, pamphlets, and articles. Will respond to questions by phone or mail.

Greenpeace
1436 U Street, NW
Washington, DC 20003
(202) 462-1177
An international organization dedicated to a wide variety of environmental issues.

Human Ecology Action League (HEAL)
P.O. Box 49126
Atlanta, Georgia 30359
Provides updated information on environmental issues and alternatives. Publishes *The Human Ecologist*.

Mothers and Others for a Livable Planet (A project of the Natural Resources Defense Council
P.O. Box 96641
Washington, DC 20090
(212) 727-4474
A national organization advocating reforms to reduce toxic exposures.

National Center for Environmental Health Strategies
1100 Rural Avenue
Voorhees, NJ 08043
(609) 429-5358
Tracks the latest scientific research and legislative, medical, legal, disability, and policy issues and publishes this information in its newsletter, *The Delicate Balance*. Also offers support services for those with environmentally- and occupationally-induced illnesses.

National Coalition Against Misuse of Pesticides (NCAMP)
530 7th Street, SE
Washington, DC 20003
Provides information assistance by both mail and phone. Advocates pesticide reform in front of senate hearings; researches and publishes information about pesticides.

Northwest Coalition for Alternatives to Pesticides (NCAP)
P.O. Box 1393
Eugene, OR 97440
Provides assistance in developing policies to protect the environment; pest management policies in schools, on roadsides, and in natural forests; and information on hundreds of pesticides and alternatives.

FREE INFORMATION ON PESTICIDES

Pesticide Hotline
(800) 858-PEST

FREE INFORMATION ON NON-√TOXIC CLEANING

Environmental Health Watch
4115 Bridge Avenue, Room 104
Cleveland, OH 44113
To receive its publication "Alternatives to Hazardous Household Chemicals and How to Dispose of Toxic Household Materials," send a self-addressed, stamped envelope.

Greenpeace
1436 U Street NW
Washington, DC 20007
(202) 462-1177
"Stepping Lightly on the Earth: Everyone's Guide to Toxics in the Home."

FREE INFORMATION ABOUT LEAD (from the Lead Protection Program)

Center for Environmental Health
Maryland Department for the Environment
2500 Broening Highway
Baltimore, MD 21224
(301) 631-3859

√RESOURCE PEOPLE

Dr. Bertram Carnow
Carnow, Conivear and Associates
20 Wacker Drive
Chicago, IL 60606
(312) 782-4486
Offers information about hazardous art materials.

Mary Oetzel
3202 West Anderson Lane, #208-249
Austin, TX 78757
(512) 288-2369
Offers on-site and phone consultations for making homes, schools, and businesses environmentally safe.

Ken Ogwaro
15022 Calle Jaunito
San Diego, CA 92129
(619) 672-0165
An entomologist and president of Ecocare, a nontoxic pest control company. Available for phone consultation to assist persons in finding nontoxic pest control products and/or organizations and companies for assistance.

TESTING

Air Quality Research Inc
901 Grayson St.
Berkeley, CA 94710
Tests for formaldehyde.

Environmental Measurements Lab
U.S. Department of Energy
376 Hudson St.
New York, NY 10014
Tests for radon.

Safe Computing Company
368 Hillside Avenue
Needham, MA 02194
(800) 222-3003
Offers the Safe Meter, a low cost instrument to measure both the magnetic component of 60 Hz fields as well as the 1,500 Hz (VLF) fields (associated with VDTs and televisions).

Safe Environments & Office Testing Service
(415) 549-9693 Available for on-site and telephone consultation for various indoor problems. Service helps identify problems such as asbestos, carbon monoxide, electromagnetic fields, formaldehyde, lead in plumbing and paint, radon, and water quality.

Watercheck/National Testing Laboratories, Inc.
6151 Wilson Mills Rd.
Cleveland, Ohio 44143
Tests for water contaminants.

APPENDIX 3

School Pesticide Survey

[Note: The following survey can be submitted to school and/or district personnel to complete regarding the previous school year; the information should then be made available to parents]

1. Which insecticides were used? How often? How much was used in a typical application?
2. Which fungicides were used? How often? How much was used in a typical application?
3. Which herbicides were used? How often? How much was used in a typical application?
4. Which rodenticides were used? How often? How much was used in a typical application?
5. Was pest control implemented by the school district or contracted out to a private company?
6. If a private company was used, how did the school monitor the application?
7. What safety precautions were implemented during and after chemical applications?
8. Before chemical applications were used, were non-chemical alternatives tried first? If not, why?
9. Were parents notified of chemical applications? If not, why?
10. Were warning signs posted after applications? If not, why?

A P P E N D I X 4

School Toxicology Information Sheet*

(Note: School and/or district personnel can be asked to complete this sheet for every chemical listed in the School Pesticide Survey, Appendix 3.)

Name of chemical _____
Class of chemical _____

Please supply what information and studies have been made available regarding the toxicity of (name of chemical) and the following areas of concern.

Cancer

Birth defects

Genetic damage

Reproductive effects

Chronic illness

Central nervous system damage

Persistence on plants, in soil, and in water

Acute toxicity

If no study has been done, please indicate so.

*Adapted from *Planning for Non-Chemical School Ground Maintenance*, Northwest Coalition for Alternatives to Pesticides, P.O. Box 13393, Eugene, Oregon, 97440

A P P E N D I X   5

Developing a Plumbing Profile of Your School*

1. When was the school built?
2. After the construction of the original building, were any new buildings or additions added? If so, when?
3. If built since December 1986, was lead-free plumbing and solder used in accordance with the lead ban?
4. When were the most recent plumbing repairs made?
5. What is the service connector made of?
6. What are the pipes made of? (Note the locations)

   copper   plastic
   galvanized metal   lead
   other   brass

7. What materials does the solder connecting the pipes contain? (Note locations with lead solder)
8. Are brass fittings, fixtures, faucets, or valves used in the drinking water system?
9. How many of the following outlets provide water for consumption? (Note the location of each)

   water coolers   drinking fountains
   ice makers   kitchen faucets
   other

10. What brands and models of water coolers are used in the school?
11. Do the faucets have accessible screens?
12. Have these screens been cleaned?
13. Are there any signs of corrosion, such as frequent leaks, rust-colored water, or stained dishes or laundry?
14. Is any electrical equipment "grounded" to water pipes? (Note their locations)
15. Have there been complaints that the drinking water tastes metallic?
16. When were water samples from the building last tested for contaminants?

    Was lead found?
    At what concentration?
    What was the pH level?
    Is testing done regularly?

17. Who supplies the school's drinking water?
    A. If purchased:
        Does the water system have any lead piping?
        How corrosive is the water?
        Is the water supply being treated now?
    B. If the school supplies its own water:
        Is the water supply treated to reduce corrosivity?
        If so, what type of treatment is used?
        Is the water treated for any purpose other than corrosion control?
        If so, for what?

[Note: The interpretation and significance of answers to this questionnaire are discussed in depth in the booklet "Lead in School Drinking Water." This booklet can be purchased from:

Superintendent of Documents
U.S. Government Printing Office
Washington, D.C. 20402

* Survey taken from: "Lead in School Drinking Water" Prepared by:

The Office of Drinking Water
Office of Water, and the United States
Environmental Protection Agency (EPA)

APPENDIX 6

Workplace Questionnaire

Use the following questionnaire to determine if you are exposed to chemicals at work that may be affecting the health of you or your family.

I. IDENTIFICATION OF CHEMICALS

Check any of the chemicals, vapors, solvents, etc., listed below that you come in direct contact with by breathing or touching while on the job.

FUMES and DUST
☐ Asbestos
☐ Plastic fumes
☐ Welding fumes
☐ Glass (e.g., Fiberglass)
☐ Silica (e.g., Sand)
☐ Plaster
☐ Other_____

ELEMENTS and METALS
☐ Aluminum
☐ Arsenic
☐ Cadmium
☐ Chromium
☐ Copper
☐ Lead
☐ Mercury
☐ Nickel
☐ Zinc
☐ Other_____

SOLVENTS
☐ Alcohols (e.g., Methyl)
☐ Benzene
☐ Toluene
☐ Xylene
☐ Carbon Tetrachloride
☐ Paint, Varnish
☐ Tetrachloroethylene
☐ Other_____

ADDITIONAL CHEMICALS
☐ Acids
☐ Detergent and Soaps
☐ Dyes
☐ Formaldehyde
☐ Pesticides (including workplaces
    serviced by pest control
    companies)
☐ Plastic resins
☐ Other_____

251

RADIATION
Check if you are exposed to one or both of the following:
□ Ionizing Radiation (e.g., X-ray)
□ Nonionizing Radiation (e.g., microwave)

II. CHEMICAL ASSESSMENT

Which chemicals are you exposed to daily?

What information do you have on the health effects of these chemicals?

Which chemicals are you exposed to periodically?

What information do you have on the acute and chronic health effects of these chemicals?

Are any of these chemicals considered carcinogens?

Are any of these chemicals considered mutagens?

Are any of these chemicals considered teratogens?

If reproductive toxins have been identified, are both sexes affected?

III. TRAINING

Recall initial and/or on-the-job training in safety to answer the following questions.

Were you ever given job safety or health training? If so, by whom? If not, why?

Have you ever received any information on the possible health effects of chemicals used on the job?

IV. PROTECTION

Answer the following questions to assess whether adequate protection is provided.

Do you wear special work clothes? If so, why?

Do you wear special work shoes? If so, why?

Is the lunchroom away from work exposures?

Are you required to wear any of the following at work: mask respirator, air supply respirator, gloves, coveralls or aprons, safety glasses, hearing protection?

If yes, how often do your wear the protection?

How often do you think the protective covering/clothing should be worn? Is this consistent with what is implemented?

V. EVALUATION

Are you satisfied that you have accurate information about the chemicals used on the job?

Are you satisfied that you have accurate information about the chemicals used in the building materials and furnishings of your workplace?

Are you satisfied that your workplace has proper ventilation?

Are you satisfied that you are protected from any potential health hazards?

Are you satisfied that any future offspring will not be jeopardized by your current work exposures?

APPENDIX 7

Listing of Chemicals under Study for Reproductive Hazards*

acetaldehyde
acrylamide
acrylic acid
acrylonitrile
Agent Orange
aldrin
aniline
arsenic
arsenic (penta-and tri-oxides)
benzene
benzo(a)pyrene
bromide, sodium
butadiene, 1,3-
butanol (butyl alcohol)
cadmium
caffeine
carbaryl
carbon dioxide
carbon disulfide
carbon monoxide
carbon tetrachloride
cellosolve, ethyl
cellosolve, methyl
chlordane
chloride
chloroform
chloroprene,B-

chromium trioxide
DDT
diazepam
dibenzofurans
dibromochloropropane
dichlorvos (aka"DDVP)
dieldrin
diethyl ether
diethylstilbestrol (DES)
dimethyl sulfoxide (DMSO)
dimethylacetamide
dimethylformamide, N,N- (DMF)
dinitroluene
diphenylamine
EDTA
epichlorohydrin
ethanol (ethyl alcohol)
ethylene dibromide
ethylene dichloride
ethylene oxide
fluorocarbon-22
furfural
glycol, ethylene
glycol, propylene
halothane
hexachlorophene
halothane

* Adapted from *JAMA*, June 1985, Vol. 253, No. 23

hexachlorophene
hydantoin
hydrazine, monohydrate
hydrofluoric acid
hydroquinone
Kepone
lead
lead, tetraethyl
lindane
lithium carbonate
lithium chloride
malathion
maleic anhydride
marijuana.
mercuric chloride
mercury
methacrylate, butyl
methacrylates
methanol
methyl iodide
methylethyl ketone
naphthalene
nickel
nitrobenzene
nitrogen dioxide
ozone
paraquat
parathion
pentachlorophenol

phthalate, dibutyl
phthalate, dimethyl
phthalic anhydride
phthalimide
piperidine, N-formyl
polybrominated biphenyls (PCBs)
propiolactone, B-
resoricinol
rotenone
selenium
styrene
sulfur dioxide
2,4 -D
2,4,5-T
TCDD, 2,3, 7,8-
thiourea methyl parathionTMTDS
tobacco
toluene
toluene diisocyanate
toluenediamine
toluidine, ortho-
toxaphene
trichlorethylene
trichloromethane
trimethyl phosphate
turpentine
urethane
vinyl chloride
xylene

APPENDIX 8

The Baby's Room Questionnaire

Directions: Answer each of the questions below. For each positive response, record the points listed at the end of the question on another piece of paper. Add up all points when finished.

1. Is the garage connected to the home? (5 points)

2. Is the baby's room directly above the garage and/or near a shared wall or entrance? (15 points)

3. Is the room carpeted with synthetic carpet? (20 points)

4. Was new carpet installed within the last six months? (25 points)

5. Is there new furniture in the room? (Award 10 points for each piece)

6. Is there any furniture made of pressed wood in the room? (Award 15 points for each piece)

7. Is the room wallpapered? (15 points)

8. Was the room wallpapered within the last six months? (15 points)

9. Has the room been painted (within the last year) with anything other than non-toxic paint? (25 points)

10. Is the crib mattress made out of synthetic fibers? (20 points)

11. Is the crib bedding made out of synthetic fibers? (20 points)

12. Are there new stuffed animals and toys in the room? (Award 5 points for each one)

Scoring:
Your baby's chances for a healthy start are the best in a room that has a score of zero. If you answered yes to all of the questions, your score could be between 200 and 250. Parents will have to decide what number is an acceptable score for their infant's room.

257

NOTES

Chapter Two

1. Lawrie Mott and Karen Snyder, *Pesticide Alert: A Guide to Pesticides in Fruits and Vegetables* (San Francisco: Sierra Club, 1987).
2. Nina Groutage and Lois Yoshishige, *Pesticide Information Packet* (Eugene, OR: Northwest Coalition for Alternatives to Pesticides, 1984).
3. Joseph Morgan, M.D. "Health Effects of Herbicides," *Human Ecologist* 7 (February 1983).
4. Mott and Snyder, *Pesticide Alert.*
5. David Weir and Mark Shapiro, *Circle of Poison: Pesticides and People in a Hungry World* (San Francisco: Institute for Food and Development Policy, 1981).
6. Anne Tattersall, "Is EPA Registration a Guarantee of Pesticide Safety?" *Journal of Pesticide Reform* (Spring 1986).
7. Anne Witt Garland, *For Our Kids' Sake* (New York: National Resources Defense Council, 1989).
8. Mary Obrien, "But What About the Other Half? The Fascinating Tale of the (Non)Inerts," *Journal of Pesticide Reform* (Summer 1986).
9. Tattersall, "EPA Registration."
10. Obrien, "(Non)Inerts."
11. Mary Obrien, "Industrial Protection Agency," *NCAP News* (Spring/Summer 1983).
12. Michael McCauley, "Contaminated Classrooms: An Investigation of Pest Control Practices of Washington, D.C., Area Schools," Washington, D.C., September 1988.
13. Mothers and Others for Pesticide Limits, *Truly Loving Care* (newsletter) 1, no. 1 (Winter 1990).

Chapter Three

1. Debra Dadd, *The Nontoxic Home* (Los Angeles: Jeremy P. Tarcher, 1986).
2. Carolyn Rueben, "Warning: Your Home May Be Hazardous to Your Health," *EastWest Magazine* 19, no. 7 (July 1989).
3. Rueben, "Warning."
4. Rueben, "Warning."
5. Dadd, *Nontoxic Home.*
6. Judith Berns, "The Cosmetic Cover-up," *Human Ecologist* 43 (Fall 1989).
7. John Elkington, *The Green Consumer* (New York: Penguin Books, 1990).
8. *The Inside Story: A Guide to Indoor Air Quality* (Washington, D.C.: United States Environmental Protection Agency, United States Consumer Product Safety Commission, 1988).

Chapter Four

1. Mott and Snyder, *Pesticide Alert.*
2. John Robbins, *Diet for a New America* (Walpole, NH: Stillpoint International, 1987).
3. Gary Null and Steven Null, *How to Get Rid of the Poisons in Your Body* (New York: Arco Publishing, 1977).
4. Dadd, *Nontoxic Home.*
5. Robbins, *Diet.*
6. Null and Null, *Poisons.*
7. Debra Dadd, *Nontoxic and Natural* (Los Angeles: Jeremy P. Tarcher, 1984).
8. Frank Oski, M.D., *Don't Drink Your Milk* (Syracuse, NY: Mollica Press, 1983).
9. Robbins, *Diet.*
10. Dadd, *Nontoxic Home.*
11. Louise Kosta, "The Sad Legacy of Lead," *Human Ecologist* 47 (Fall 1990).
12. Mott and Snyder, *Pesticide Alert.*

Chapter Five

1. Null and Null, *Poisons.*
2. Phyllis Saifer, M.D., M.P.H., and Merla Zellerback, *Detox* (New York: Ballentine Books, 1984).
3. "Fifty Years of Declining Fertility," *EastWest Magazine* (December 1990).
4. Robbins, *Diet.*
5. "Declining Fertility."
6. Ruth Heifeitz and Sharon Taylor, "Mother's Milk or Mother's Poison?" *Journal of Pesticide Reform* 9, no. 3 (Fall 1989).
7. Heifeitz and Taylor, "Mother's Poison,"
8. F. Weiner, *Journal of Pediatrics* (September 1979).
9. Dadd, *Nontoxic and Natural.*
10. Irving Selifoff, *Health Hazards of Asbestos* (New York: Annals of the New York Academy of Science).

Chapter Six

1. Newsletter from National Jewish Center for Immunology and Respiratory Medicine, 20 August 1990.
2. Sherry Rogers, M.D. *Tired or Toxic?* (Syracuse, NY: Prestige Publishing, 1990).
3. William Crook, M.D., "Hyperactivity and Attention Deficit Disorder—Old and New Perspectives," *Human Ecologist* (Winter 1990).
4. Rogers, *Tired or Toxic.*
5. "In Japan, Fast Food is Fast Becoming a Health Hazard," *Chicago Tribune*, 14 October 1990.
6. Debra Dadd, *Nontoxic, Natural and Earthwise* (Los Angeles: Jeremy P. Tarcher, 1990).
7. Oski, *Don't Drink Your Milk.*
8. Rapp, *Impossible Child.*

9. Dennis Remington, *Back to Health* (Provo, UT: Vitality House International, 1986).

10. Rapp, *Impossible Child.*

11. Rapp, *Impossible Child.*

BIBLIOGRAPHY

"Alternatives to Toxic Termite Control." San Diego: Environmental Health Coalition.

Baier, Edward. "Endangered Species." *Occupational Health and Safety* (July 1987).

Banta, John. "A Shopper's Guide to Electromagnetic Field Monitor." *East West* (May 1990).

Beaudry, Anne. "Biodegradable Diapers: A Pseudo Solution. *Mothering* 53 (Fall 1989).

Becker, Robert O. "Electromagnetic Fields: What You Can Do." *East West* (May 1990).

Begley, Sharon and Mary Hayer. "A Guide to the Grocery." *Newsweek* 27 March 1989.

Berns, Judith. "An Interview with Dr. Randolph." *Human Ecologist* 43 (Fall 1989).

Berns, Judith. "The Cosmetic Cover-up." *Human Ecologist* 43 (Fall 1989).

Bond, Anne Berthold. *Clean and Green: The Complete Guide to Nontoxic and Environmentally Safe Housekeeping.* Woodstock, NY: Ceres Publishing, 1990.

Bower, John. "The Floor Plan for Health." *EastWest* 19, no. 7 (July 1989).

"ChemLawn Yields in New York Suit." *Pesticides and You* 10, no. 3 (August 1990).

Chicago Tribune, 14 October 1990.

"Chlordane Contaminated School Shut." *Pesticides and You* 9, no. 3 (August 1989).

"Contaminated Mother's Milk." *Human Ecologist* 35 (1987).

Crook, William, M.D. *Tracking Down Hidden Food Allergies.* Jackson, TN: Professional Books, 1978.

Crook, William, M.D. *The Yeast Connection.* New York: Random House, 1986.

Dadd, Debra. *Nontoxic and Natural.* Los Angeles: Jeremy P. Tarcher, 1984.

Dadd, Debra. *The Nontoxic Home.* Los Angeles: Jeremy P. Tarcher, 1986.

Dadd, Debra. *Nontoxic, Natural, and Earthwise.* Los Angeles: Jeremy P. Tarcher, 1990.

Davidhoff, Linda Lee. "Multiple Chemical Sensitivities (MCS)." *Amicus Journal* (Winter 1989).

"Diazinon Spraying Causes Evacuation." *Pesticides and You* 9, no. 4 (October 1989).

"The Dioxin Connection." *Mothering* 53 (Fall 1989).

"Drugs in Livestock and Poultry Feed: Human Health Effects." *Human Ecologist* (Winter 1985-86).

Duffy, William. *Suger Blues.* New York: Warner Books, 1976.

"Effects of Toxic Chemicals on the Reproductive System." Council on Scientific Affairs. *JAMA* 253, no. 23, 21 June 1985.

Elkington, John, Julia Hailes and Joel Makower. *The Green Consumer.* New York: Penguin Books, 1990.

Garland, Anne Witt. *For Our Kids' Sake*. New York: National Resources Defense Council, 1989.

Golos, Natalie and Frances Golbitz. *Coping With Your Allergies*. New York: Simon and Schuster, 1979.

Groutage, Nina and Lois Yoshishige. *Pesticide Information Packet*. Eugene, OR: Northwest Coalition for Alternatives to Pesticides, 1984.

Heifetz, Ruth and Sharon Taylor. "Mother's Milk or Mother's Poison?" *Journal of Pesticide Reform* 9, no. 3 (Fall 1989).

Hollis, Robert. "The Ethics of Diapering." *Mothering* 53 (Fall 1989).

Hormann, Elizabeth. "New Breast-feeding Challenges." *Mothering* 53 (Fall 1989).

Hunter, Beatrice Trum. "Diet and Health for Children." *Human Ecologist* (Fall 1990).

The Inside Story: A Guide to Indoor Air Quality. Washington, DC: United States Environmental Protection Agency, United States Consumer Product Safety Commission, 1988.

Kosta, Loiuse. "Electromagnetic Fields: Unanswered Questions." *Human Ecologist* (Winter 1990).

Kosta, Louise. "The Sad Legacy of Lead." *Human Ecologist* (Fall 1990).

Jacobson, Lauren. *Children's Art Hazards*. New York: The Natural Resources Defense Council.

Lappe, Frances Moore. *Diet for a Small Planet*. New York: Ballantine Books, 1982.

Lawson, Lynn. "Hospitals and Nursing Homes: A Special Need." *Human Ecologist* (Fall 1989).

Lead in School Drinking Water. Washington, DC: Office of Drinking Water, Office of Water, United States Environmental Protection Agency, 1989.

"Letter to Members." Northwest Coalition for Alternatives to Pesticides, 1989.

Lifton, Bernice. *Bug Busters: Getting Rid of Household Pests Without Dangerous Chemicals*. New York: McGraw Hill Book Company, 1985.

Lipkin, Janet. "Treating Head Lice: It's a Pesticide Issue, Too." *Journal of Pesticide Reform* 9, no. 3 (Fall 1989).

Lohmeier, Lynne, Ph.D. "Make Work Safe for Childbearing Couples." *East West* 17, no. 8 (August 1987).

Lowengart, Ruth A. "Childhood Leukemia and Parents of Occupational and Home Exposures." *JNCI* 79 (July 1987).

Marchi, Louis. "Secret Inert Ingredients Compound Pesticide Toxicities." *Human Ecologist* (Spring 1990).

Mason, Jim. "Dairy Drugs." *Vegetarian Times*. (June 1990).

Mayell, Mark. "Zap Control." *EastWest* (May 1990).

McCarty, Meredith. *American Macrobiotic Cuisine*. Eureka, CA: Turning Point Publications, 1986.

McCauley, Michael. "Contaminated Classrooms: An Investigation of Pest Control Practices of Washington, DC Area Schools." (September 1988).

McEntire, Patricia. *Mommy—I'm Hungry*. Sacramento: Couger Books, 1985.

Mead, Mark N. "Chlorination: Friend or Foe?" *East West* (December 1989).

Morgan, Joseph, M.D. "Health Effects of Herbicides." *Human Ecologist* 7 (February 1983).

Mott, Lawrie. "Pesticides in Food: Your Daily Dose." *Northwest Coalition for Alternatives to Pesticides News* (Spring/Summer 1983).

Mott, Lawrie and Karen Snyder. *Pesticide Alert: A Guide to Pesticides in Fruits and Vegetables*. San Francisco: Sierra Club, 1987.

Mueller, William. "Testing Your Tap Water." *East West* (June 1990).

National Jewish Center for Immunology and Respiratory Medicine. (letter) 20 August 1990.

Newman, Penny. "Cancer Clusters Among Children: The Implications of McFarland." *Journal of Pesticide Reform* 9, no. 3 (Fall 1989).

"News You Can Use." *Bio-talks* 16 (May/June 1989).

Null, Gary and Steven Null. *How to Get Rid of the Poisons in Your Body*. New York: Arco Publishing, 1977.

Obrien, Mary. "But What About the Other Half? The Fascinating Tale of the (Non)Inerts." *Journal of Pesticide Reform* (Summer 1986).

Obrien, Mary. "Round-up/Glyphosate." Northwest Coalition for Alternatives to Pesticides.

Obrien, Mary. "Diazinon." Northwest Coalition for Alternatives to Pesticides.

Obrien, Mary. "Industrial Protection Agency." *Northwest Coalition for Alternatives to Pesticides News* (Spring/Summer 1983).

Oetzel, Mary. "Build for Health." *Human Ecologist* 21 (Spring 1983).

Oski, Frank, M.D. *Don't Drink Your Milk*. Syracuse: Mollica Press, 1983.

Pimental, David. "Benefits and Costs of Pesticide Use in U.S. Food Production." *Northwest Coalition for Alternatives to Pesticides News* (Spring/Summer 1982).

Pitman, Sue. "A Landmark Ordinance in Waucondo, Illinois." *Northwest Coalition for Alternatives to Pesticides News* (Spring/Summer 1984).

Planning for Non-Chemical School Maintenance. Eugene, OR: Northwest Coalition for Alternatives to Pesticides.

Plunkett, Julie. "Natural Nontoxic Pest Control." *Ocean Beach Natural Foods Co-op News*. (August/September 1990).

"Protecting Against Salmonella." *Truly Loving Care Newsletter* (Mothers and Others for Pesticide Limits, New York) 2, no. 1 (Winter 1990).

"Radon, an Environmental Concern." *Human Ecologist* (Winter 1985-86).

Rapp, Doris, M.D. *The Impossible Child*. Buffalo, NY: Practical Allergy Research Foundation, 1986.

Rea, William J., M.D. "Sick Building Syndrome." *Human Ecologist* (Summer 1990).

Reproductive Hazards in the Workplace. Washington, DC: Office of Technology Assessment/Congressional Board of the 99th Congress, 1985.

Reuben, Carolyn. "Warning: Your Home May Be Hazardous to Your Health." *East West* 19, no. 7 (July 1989).

Robbins, John. *Diet for a New America*. Walpole, NH: Stillpoint Publishing, 1987.

Rogers, Sherry A., M.D. "The Sick School Syndrome." *Human Ecologist*. (Fall 1988).

Rogers, Sherry A., M.D. *Tired or Toxic?* Syracuse: Prestige Publishing, 1990.

Rousseau, David and W. J. Rea. *Your Home, Health, and Well-Being*. Berkeley: Ten Speed Press, 1988.

Saifer, Phyllis, M.D., M.P.H., and Merla Zellerbach. *Detox*. New York: Ballantine Books, 1984.

Schmidt, Michael A. *Childhood Ear Infections: What Every Parent and Physician Should Know.* Berkeley: North Atlantic Books, 1990.

Selikoff, Irving J. and E. Cuyler Hammond. *Health Hazards of Asbestos Exposure.* New York: Annals of the New York Academy of Science, 1979.

Sellin, Mary. "The Mythology of Pesticide Safety." *Northwest Coalition for Alternatives to Pesticides News.* (Spring/Summer 1983).

"Skin Absorption: An Important Route of Exposure." *Toxinformer* (Environmental Health Coalition, San Diego) (May/June 1989).

Tattersall, Ann. "Is EPA Registration a Guarantee of Pesticide Safety?" *Journal of Pesticide Reform* (Spring 1986).

"Testing Your Home Pesticide Residues." *Human Ecologist* 35 (1987).

Thomson, Bill. "Health Hazards in the Workplace." *East West* 17, no. 8 (August 1987).

"Toward a Chlorine-free Pulp and Paper Industry." *Greenpeace Action/Toxics* (Washington DC) 1989.

Truly Loving Care Newsletter (Mothers and Others for Pesticide Limits, New York) 1, no. 1 (Winter 1990).

Turner, Kristina *Self-Healing Cookbook.* Grass Valley, CA: Earthtone Press, 1987.

Ubell, Earl. "One Lump or Two?" *Parade Magazine,* 12 November 1989.

Weir, David and Mark Shapiro. *Circle of Poison: Pesticides and People in a Hungry World.* San Francisco: Institute for Food and Development Policy, 1981.

Weiss, Linda. "Toxins in the Classroom." *Human Ecologist* (Fall 1990).

"Why Take 'Cides? Alternatives Work." San Diego: Environmental Health Coalition.

Zamm, Alfred. *Why Your House May Endanger Your Health.* New York: Simon and Schuster, 1980.

INDEX

ABOUT THE AUTHOR

As an educator and author of innovative educational programs used in schools nationwide, Nancy Sokol Green's work has always focused on children with special needs. However, after discovering that she had become critically ill from common, everyday chemical exposures, she now believes that there may be another group of children with special needs—those with learning problems, negative behaviors, and ill-health which may unknowingly be triggered by exposures to daily chemicals. Because the possibility of a chemical/health connection may not yet be evident to many educators and parents, she is motivated to bring this awareness to as many individuals as possible.

She presently lives with her husband and two daughters in Carlsbad, California.